Osseous Reconstruction of the Maxilla and the Mandible

Philip J. Boyne

Osseous Reconstruction of the Maxilla and the Mandible: Surgical Techniques Using Titanium Mesh and Bone Mineral

Philip J. Boyne, DMD, MS, DSc (hon)
Professor of Oral & Maxillofacial Surgery
School of Dentistry
Loma Linda University
Loma Linda, California

With a contribution by Michael Peetz, PhD
Director, Biomaterials Division
Geistlich Sons, Ltd
Wolhusen, Switzerland

Quintessence Publishing Co, Inc
Chicago, Berlin, London, Tokyo, São Paulo, Moscow, Prague and Warsaw

To Mary Anne,

for a half century of love, grace, patience, and support.

Library of Congress Cataloging-In-Publication Data

Boyne, Philip J.
    Osseous reconstruction of the maxilla and the mandible: surgical techniques using titanium mesh and bone mineral / Philip J. Boyne: with a contribution by Michael Peetz.
        p.   cm.
    Includes bibliographical references and index.
    ISBN 0-86715-319-9
    1. Maxilla—Surgery. 2. Mandible—Surgery. 3. Bone-grafting.
4. Titanium—Therapeutic use. 5. Wire netting—Therapeutic use.
I. Peetz, Michael. II. Title.
    [DNLM: 1. Maxilla—surgery. 2. Mandible—surgery. 3. Bone Transplantation—methods. 4. Surgical Mesh. 5. Titanium.
6. Implants, Artificial. WU 610 B793o 1996]
RK529.B69 1996
617.5'2059—dc20
DNLM/DLC   96-26147
for Library of Congress   CIP

© 1997 by Quintessence Publishing Co, Inc

Published by Quintessence Publishing Co, Inc
551 N. Kimberly Drive
Carol Stream, IL 60188

All rights reserved. This book or any part thereof may not be reproduced, stored in a retrieval system, or transmitted in any form or by any means, electronic, mechanical, photocopying, recording, or otherwise, without prior written permission of the publisher.

Editor: Lane Evensen
Production: Timothy M. Robbins

Printed in Hong Kong

Contents

Preface vii

Acknowledgments viii

Introduction ix

Part I. Bone Grafts

1. Bone Grafts: Materials 3
2. Bone Grafts: Mechanisms 13

Part II. Surgical Reconstruction Using Titanium Mesh in Combination with Bone Grafts

3. For Restoration with Conventional Prostheses 25
4. For Restoration with Root-Form Implants 37
5. After Combination Syndrome, Trauma, or Oncologic Surgery 53
6. For Treatment of Maxillary Clefts 75

Appendix: Characterization of Xenogeneic Bone Material 87

Index 101

Preface

Successful evaluation of patients' bone deficits and defects and the relation of this clinical assessment to the implementation of effective prosthodontic systems to produce functional reconstruction has been a major clinical problem for some time. The selection of an appropriate bone graft material, and the application of the most effective oral and maxillofacial surgical augmentation techniques are the extremely important treatment approaches that logically follow the assessment of the clinical extent and the anatomic nature of the host bone sites.

The concepts discussed in this text and the techniques described bring about a quality reconstruction of many types of defects of the mandible as well as the maxilla. The procedure has proven to be successful through 25 years of clinical use involving TiMesh (TiMesh, Inc, Las Vegas, NV) with particulate marrow and cancellous bone (PMCB) and 10 years involving the use of TiMesh with PMCB and Bio-Oss (Geistlich Sons, Wolhusen, Switzerland; Osteohealth Co, Shirley, NY). The final result has been one of enhanced function and esthetics, which has been extremely useful in many types of surgical prosthetic rehabilitation cases. The technique of combining a quality titanium product with a particulate marrow cancellous bone autogenous graft together with a highly conductive porous bone material conducive to increasing bone density brings about excellent results.

Since the maxilla has been a principal area of clinical concern due to the presence of the perinasal sinuses, poorly trabeculated bone, and decreased bone density in edentulous areas, a special bone grafting system was developed by us to address this problem.

This text will describe in detail the technique for the application of the surgical system using titanium mesh and particulate bone grafts. The purpose of this report is to enable the health care practitioner to use the system described in a number of different areas to effectively reconstruct those patients having severe-to-moderate bony deficiencies of the maxilla. We will be dealing with the unique anatomic characteristics presenting in the maxilla that make that particular bone area a more difficult one to restore surgically than some other areas of the jaws (eg anterior mandible). The same procedure does have application to the mandible as well, and extension of the technique to lower jaw defects will also be presented.

Additionally, the technique can be used in reconstruction of traumatic and oncologic surgical defects of the midface. As such the material presented in the work would be of interest not only to oral-maxillofacial surgeons but also to otolaryngologists and plastic and reconstructive surgeons in developing new procedures for reconstructive rehabilitation of patients with large areas of facial bone loss.

Acknowledgments

We wish to thank Robert K. Schenk, MD, Prof Dr Med, Professor Emeritus of Anatomy, Institute of Pathophysiology, University of Berne, Berne, Switzerland, for reproduction of some of his histologic material.

We acknowledge the technical assistance of June Barrientos in preparing the computerized material for this text.

Introduction

Various bone-grafting techniques have been utilized by oral and maxillofacial surgeons for the reconstruction of the maxilla and the mandible over the past three decades. Although, initially, the height and width of the bone can be restored by the use of free, nonvascularized autogenous bone grafts, these grafted areas tend to resorb under the influence of conventional prostheses. Insufficient attention has been given to the development of bone-grafting techniques that would have the end result of increasing the bone density of the restored area. It is not sufficient merely to increase the height and the width of the bony ridge; increased bone density is necessary to create a bony matrix that will resist resorption.

Bony reconstruction of the maxilla, for root-form implants as well as for conventional prostheses, requires increased bone density. The reason for this is that many parts of the maxilla, particularly in the posterior area, have decreased density as a result of osteoporotic changes and the effect of long-standing edentulism.[1] Therefore, when root-form implants are to be placed in such areas, it is desirable to use techniques that will restore density to the bone and that will resist resorption over the long term.

One of the most efficient methods of accomplishing this objective is to combine osteoconductive, slowly resorbing, calcified bone graft substitutes with autogenous particulate marrow and cancellous bone. In such a system, the target cells in the autogenous marrow are available for induction to form new bone while the conductive effect is provided by the bone substitute portion of the graft.

The conductive effect of a slowly remodeling bone graft substitute tends to maintain an increased bone density over a long period of time.[2] Materials that are not remodeled at all and materials on the other end of the spectrum, which are resorbed and disappear within a few days or a few weeks, should not be used. Thus, porous bone mineral, such as Bio-Oss (Geistlich Sons/Osteohealth Co), is an excellent material to use to effect the desired result.

In our studies utilizing porous bone mineral with particulate marrow and cancellous autogenous bone, we have found in mature rhesus monkeys that there has been an increased bone density 1.5 years after grafting in the area of the root-form implants.[1] Additionally, in clinical studies, increased bone density and lack of resorption have been observed under conventional prostheses when porous bone mineral has been used appropriately with an autograft.[2]

In the very near future, bone-inductive materials bioengineered through the use of recombinant DNA will introduce a new era, enabling the surgeon to induce bone formation and repair with an appropriate carrier for the bone-inductive material. The same carrier could also be used as an osteoconductive material to effect a slow resorption and remodeling process to increase bone density. Thus, the initial bone formation and the long-term osseous remodeling could be effected by the same material if the appropriate system is carefully selected.

In the future, bone-inductive materials (recombinant human bone morphogenetic protein [rhBMP]) with appropriate carriers and conductors will be used to effect a long-term increased bone density. For the present, it is through the application of an appropriate conductive material (Bio-Oss), the possible use of guided tissue regeneration membranes and barriers, and the employment of titanium mesh to initially maintain the appropriate contour and position of the graft in the deficient area that the optimal osseous reconstruction for maxillary and mandibular implant-borne prostheses may be achieved.

References

1. Boyne PJ. Analysis of performance of root-form endosseous implants placed in the maxillary sinus. J Long-Term Effects Med Implants 1993;3:143–159.
2. Boyne PJ. Vergleich von Bio-Oss und anderen Implantationsmaterialien bei der Erhaltung des Alveolarkammes des Unterkiefers beim Menschen. Unfallheilkunde 1991;216:98–103.

Part I
Bone Grafts

Chapter 1

Bone Grafts: Materials

The types of grafts available for the maxilla and mandible are the autogenous, allogeneic, alloplastic, and xenogeneic. *Autogenous* grafts are taken from the same person.[1] *Allogeneic* grafts are composed of tissues taken from another individual of the same species. *Alloplastic* materials are synthetic substances used as substitutes for bone in grafting, and *xenogeneic* grafts are composed of tissue taken from another species (ie, from an animal source, usually bovine).

Autogenous Bone

Autogenous grafts are usually harvested from one of the following donor sites:

1. Iliac crest (anterior superior crest or posterior superior crest)
2. Rib
3. Calvaria
4. Anterior tibia
5. Intraoral sites
6. Free flaps (eg, fibula with microvascular anastomosis)

The principal harvesting sources of bone-grafting materials are selected primarily to provide the maximal amount of particulate marrow and cancellous bone (PMCB) to deliver the highest potential number of pluripotential or osteogenic precursor cells[2] in the graft material mass. These cells are used in effecting the restoration of the deficient bone area. Although some pluripotential cells exist in the host bone wall, depending on the type of defect involved, delivery of a graft of high osteogenetic material with a great number of these preosteoblastic cells and pluripotential cells tends to increase the potential for success and enhance the quality of the final restorative result.[2-5] Therefore, most of the donor sites used for autogenous bone grafting provide a basis for obtaining an optimally high amount of PMCB.

The iliac crest graft is considered to be the gold standard of graft materials because of the high population of pluripotential cells in the particulate cancellous bone and marrow portion of the graft. These cells are available for induction to become osteoblasts and to form new bone. These pluripotential cells are located primarily in the vascular marrow spaces of the cancellous bone (PMCB)[5] (Figs 1-1 and 1-2).

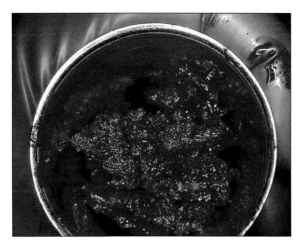

Fig 1-1 Curetted particulate marrow and cancellous bone usually used in the reconstruction of oral and maxillofacial defects, particularly around root-form implants.

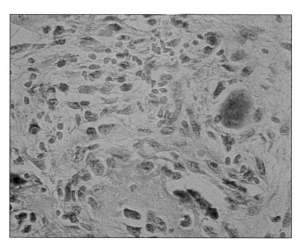

Fig 1-2 Photomicrograph of marrow vascular spaces in a particulate marrow and cancellous bone graft showing different types of cells, including the pluripotential cells, which have the ability to become osteoblasts and to form new bone (original magnification ×150).

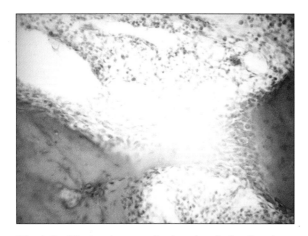

Fig 1-3 Photomicrograph showing induction in a vascular marrow space with a mass composed of many osteoblasts joining one trabecula to another. This is an excellent example of induction, in which pluripotential cells are influenced to become osteoblasts in large numbers (original magnification ×100).

The process of stimulation of these cells to become osteoblasts is called *induction*, and various inductive mechanisms can be used to stimulate pluripotential cells to become osteogenic. When this phenomenon occurs, there is a change in the morphology of the pluripotential undifferentiated cell, producing an osteoblast and the subsequent formation of bone. This phenomenon is quite remarkable and easily recognized histologically (Fig 1-3).

Among the various donor sites, the posterior iliac crest has a possibility of delivering up to 80 cm^3 of PMCB-type bone, whereas a single rib site has a very small amount of cancellous bone and marrow (Table 1-1). The calvaria likewise has a lower amount of cancellous bone. Thus, the area of choice is the posterior iliac crest, which can deliver the greatest amount of cancellous bone and marrow. The next most desirable sites, in order of preference, are the anterior iliac crest and the calvaria.

Table 1-1 Amount of particulate marrow and cancellous bone (PMCB) available from various donor sites

Sites	PMCB
Anterior iliac crest	30–50 cm^3
Posterior iliac crest	60–80 cm^3
Calvarium	20–25 cm^3
Single rib	10–15 cm^3

Sources of Bone

Ilium

Surgical Techniques for Harvesting

The initial incision should be made approximately 2 cm posterior to the anterior superior iliac spine and 1 cm inferior to the crest of the ridge. The incision is extended approximately 5 cm in length. The dissection is carried down through the fascia lata femoris. The gluteus minimus and gluteus medius muscles are detached from the aponeurosis of the crest of the ilium. After the lateral table is removed with a curved reciprocating saw or a curved chisel, the PMCB bone is curetted. After the graft is harvested, the area is irrigated well and the gluteus minimus and gluteus medius muscles are reattached to the crest of the ridge. The soft tissues are closed in layers.

Depending on the amount of bleeding from the marrow spaces at the time of closure, a drain may or may not be placed. If a drain is placed, it is always inserted in the second layer immediately superficial to the gluteus medius and gluteus minimus muscles, which have been closed to the crest of the ridge. It is usually removed on the second postoperative day. We prefer a small miniflap drain; the suction bulb is changed at 4-hour intervals during the first postoperative day.

Figures 1-4 to 1-9 show the surgical procedure for obtaining bone from the anterior iliac crest and Figs 1-10 to 1-13 show the procedure for obtaining a bone graft from the posterior iliac crest.

A trephined core of the iliac crest can be taken with an 8 to 12-mm-diameter trephine power-driven instrument (Fig 1-14). This graft consists of a combination of cortical and cancellous bone or all cortical bone. The advantage of taking this trephined core of graft material over the direct approach with curettage of the cancellous bone, however, is not great, and the technique is no longer extensively used. This technique can be carried out through a small incision and done "blindly" (Fig 1-15). However, this reduced incision technique is not recommended because of the danger of perforating both cortices with the power trephine and the difficulty of judging the depth and thickness of the iliac crest.

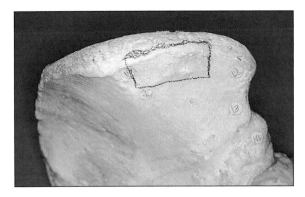

Fig 1-4 Bony crest of the ilium and the anterior superior iliac spine. The area of the lateral table, which is surgically removed to obtain PMCB for grafting, is outlined with a rectangle.

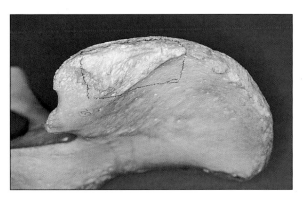

Fig 1-5 Anterior (right) and posterior (left) superior iliac spines.

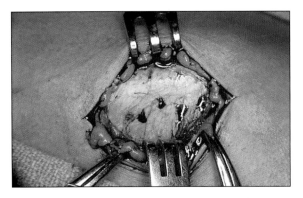

Fig 1-6 Surgical approach for harvesting of PMCB from the anterior crest of the ilium, showing retraction of skin and subcutaneous tissue.

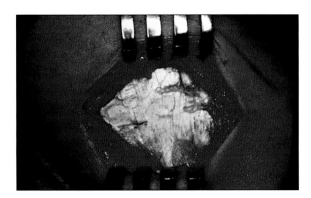

Fig 1-7 Dissection to the level of the fascial lata over the crest of the anterior iliac ridge. The fascia is covering the gluteus medius and gluteus minimus muscles.

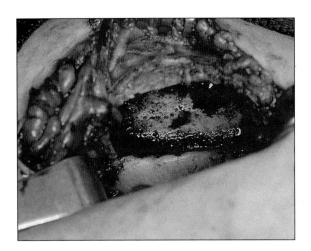

Fig 1-8 View after removal of the lateral iliac table window and curettage of the deep cancellous bone and marrow, exposing the underlying surface of the medial cortical bone table. Care is taken not to perforate the medial table, because an intact medial cortex facilitates the hemostatic management of any postoperative bleeding complication. This type of osseous defect tends to heal with good bone formation. (When other techniques, such as complete ostectomy of both bony cortices, are used, the area heals with a marked defect at the iliac crest.) The maintenance of the inner table thus facilitates good osseous regeneration of the donor site.

Sources of Bone

Fig 1-9 Suturing of the donor site. After closure of the gluteus medius muscle to the aponeurosis of the crest of the ilium, the skin is usually closed with 4-0 nylon interrupted sutures following closure of the subcutaneous tissue with 3-0 chromic sutures.

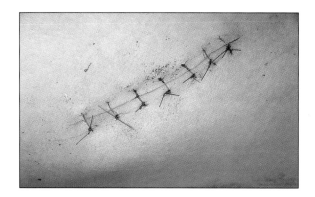

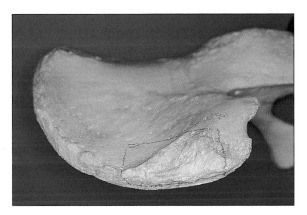

Fig 1-10 Dry specimen demonstrating the area involved with the posterior iliac crest (lower right). The crest of the posterior superior iliac spine is thicker than the anterior crest. Additional cancellous bone and marrow can be obtained from this approach, and up to 80 cm^3 of PMCB can be harvested from one posterior crest.

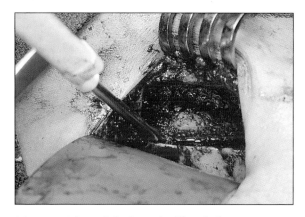

Fig 1-11 View of the lateral table window osteotomy ventral to the posterior superior iliac spine, showing the size of the cortical bone area involved. A large amount of cancellous bone and marrow can be obtained from this donor site.

Fig 1-12 Posterior superior iliac spine donor site after removal of the cancellous bone and marrow. After harvesting of the bone graft, a collagen hemostatic agent may be placed in the defect temporarily to obtain hemostasis prior to closure of the gluteus maximus and gluteus medius to the aponeurosis of the posterior crest. Muscular and fascial closure is obtained with 3-0 chromic gut suture. The final skin closure is with 4-0 nylon suture.

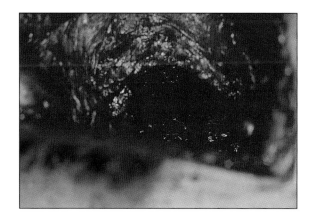

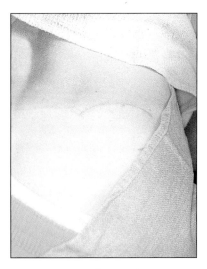

Fig 1-13 Well-healed posterior crest donor site with excellent esthetic skin closure and good functional results.

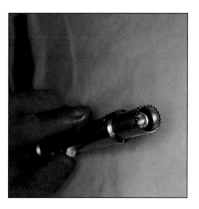

Fig 1-14 Ten-millimeter orthopedic trephine, which can be used to obtain a core of cortical-cancellous bone from the iliac crest either in a blind small-incision approach or through a larger open-incision technique.

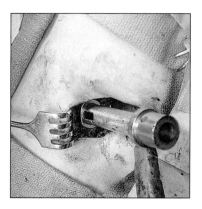

Fig 1-15 Use of a trephine to obtain a specimen of graft material from the iliac crest through a small incision.

Complications and Morbidities

The principal complications of taking bone from the posterior iliac crest are adynamic ileus and hernia. However, in reviewing more than 170 cases involving posterior iliac crest harvesting performed on our service over the past 18 years, we have not observed a single cases of ileus or bowel hernia.

Harvesting of the anterior iliac crest has been reported to be associated with paresthesia of the lateral femoral cutaneous nerve. In our experience with more than 300 anterior iliac crest donor sites, only one patient has experienced paresthesia of the lateral femoral cutaneous nerve. This complication occurs primarily when the incision is made too far inferiorly on the lateral aspect of the thigh or too far anteriorly, involving an incision immediately below the anterior iliac spine, creating an opportunity for interdiction of the lateral femoral cutaneous nerve. Thus, the harvesting of bone from the iliac crest is, in our experience, met with very little postoperative morbidity.

Patients are usually ambulated on the first postoperative day and released from the hospital on the second postoperative day (sometimes even on the first day after surgery) and are allowed to use a cane or a walker during ambulation for the first 5 days at home. Except for not being able to climb several sets of stairs, to drive an automobile, or to elevate the leg forcefully during the first postoperative week, patients experience very little restriction in their range of motion or ambulation. The patient is allowed to ambulate at will and to move slowly during the first few days postoperatively.

The principal minor complication that we have observed after this iliac crest procedure has been formation of hematomas. When a hematoma occurs following an anterior iliac crest procedure in which the medial table is allowed to remain intact, simple reapplication of a pressure dressing with or without aspiration of the hematoma or seroma suffices to treat the swelling.

If the medial table approach has been used in an anterior iliac crest harvesting procedure and a postoperative hematoma occurs, it is very difficult to reach the involved area for aspiration and also difficult to apply a pressure dressing in the correct direction to effectively control the hemorrhage. Although the medial table technique is used by many surgeons, we believe that the lateral table approach results in fewer postoperative hematomas.

If the anterior superior iliac spine is inadvertently taken in the surgical procedure, several complications can ensue. One of these is interference in the function of the sartorius muscle. This affects the patient's walking and, particularly, the patient's ability to lift and abduct the leg (in the manner of crossing the knees when sitting). There is also an increased incidence of postoperative hernia when the anterior superior iliac spine is taken. Additionally, the patient tends to experience considerable discomfort during ambulation with a full-gaited walk, experiencing a delay in final rehabilitation for a matter of 3 to 4 weeks. Therefore, we believe that the safest bone-harvesting procedure is one in which the anterior iliac crest is harvested through the lateral approach, leaving the medial table, the iliac crest itself, and the anterior superior iliac spine all intact.

Cranium

Cranial or calvarial bone grafts are usually obtained by taking the outer table of the calvarium with the underlying cancellous bone and marrow. The cortical bone of the calvarial graft may be used in one piece or morselized and mixed with the cancellous bone particles.

One problem associated with calvarial grafts is that they are composed primarily of cortical bone matrix. This property makes such a graft excellent for recontouring facial bone areas. Such a graft, however, does not have the same results when applied to the alveolar bone of the mandible and maxilla, particularly when the case involves the reconstruction of the mandible and maxilla for root-form implants. The amount of PMCB obtainable from cranial grafts is limited compared to the amount found in the iliac crest. Calvarial bone grafts, when subjected to the stress of occlusal forces through conventional prostheses or root-form, implant-borne prostheses, tend to resorb and tend not to maintain the form and contour of the reconstructed bone area.

Fibula

A fibular bone transfer, when used as a free graft with microvascular anastomosis, tends to produce a very successful soft-tissue graft transfer. However, the osseous portion of the composite graft is composed, for the most part, of thick cortical bone and as a result does not usually offer a high quantity of viable cells (Fig 1-16) for facilitating osseointegration with titanium root-form implant surfaces. In our experience, root-form implants placed in such grafts require a longer period of time for integration than do similar implants placed in PMCB-grafted areas. Once implants are well integrated, however, the result can be prosthetically satisfactory.

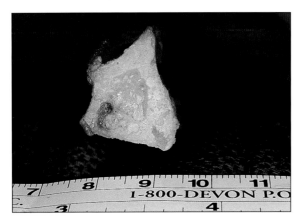

Fig 1-16 Cross section of a free fibular graft. The large amount of cortical bone and extensive central medullary canal are shown. Little cancellous bone is present. Cells of the medullary canal are maintained in a viable state by microvascular anastomosis.

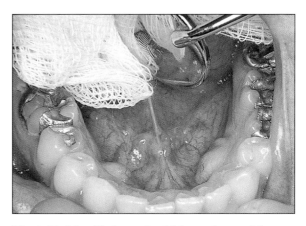

Fig 1-17 Mandibular tori, which can be used for autogenous particulate cortical grafts. Grafts taken from the tori have very little cancellous bone and so have very few pluripotential or precursor cells and a diminished capability of forming bone by cellular induction.

Anterior Tibia

The anterior tibial surface can be used also as a source for cancellous bone and marrow. A moderate amount of PMCB may be obtained from the tibia (see Table 1-1) and the procedure usually results in very little morbidity. Thus, as an alternative site for autogenous bone when approximately 30 to 40 cm^3 of PMCB is needed, the anterior tibial surface can be used preferentially after the posterior and anterior iliac crest have been considered.

Intraoral Sites

All donor sites already discussed produce PMCB graft material that can be used in reconstructing the maxilla and mandible and for the insertion of root-form implants. If small amounts of cancellous and marrow bone are needed, an intraoral source may be used. The intraoral sites most frequently used are the mentum, which contains mostly cortical bone; the area behind the mandibular third molar; mandibular tori, which also contain largely cortical bone (Fig 1-17); and the maxillary tuberosity.

The intraoral site that we prefer is the retromolar area of the mandible. This site can be entered by simply using a small, round bur to perforate the cortical bone of the anterior surface of the ascending ramus posterior to the third molar. The small cortical bone plate is elevated to expose the underlying cancellous bone, which is then curretted in a horizontal direction posteriorly into the ramus. The currette is always kept in a plane parallel to the occlusal surface of the mandibular teeth to prevent injury to the mandibular canal and the inferior alveolar nerve. There is little chance of postoperative morbidity if care is taken measuring from the anterior border of the ramus to the mandibular canal. The procedure can be used bilaterally if additional graft material is needed (Figs 1-18a to 1-18c).

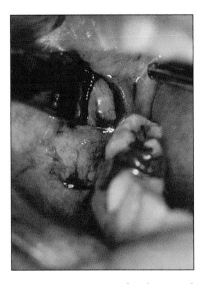 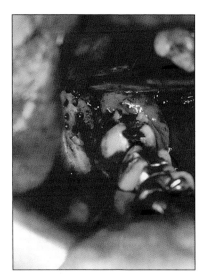 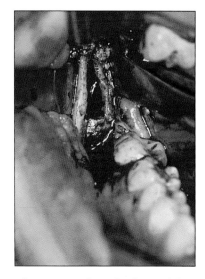

Fig 1-18a Retromolar intraoral site to be used for an autogenous graft. The incision is made along the anterior border of the ramus, and a relaxing incision is made at the distal aspect of the second molar, exposing the retromolar cortical bone.

Fig 1-18b Perforation of the cortical layer of retromolar bone with a small round bur. Bur holes are made approximately 2 mm apart.

Fig 1-18c Triangular bone defect created when the bur holes in the retromolar area are joined. Cancellous bone for grafting may be harvested from around this site by curretting posteriorly directly into the ramus.

References

1. Boyne PJ. Maxillofacial surgery. In Habal M (ed). Bone Grafts and Bone Substitutes. Philadelphia: Saunders, 1992:291–298.

2. Friedenstein AJ. Determined and inducible osteogenic precursor cells. In: Sognnaes RF (ed). Proceedings of the CIBA Foundation Symposium No. 11 on Hard Tissue Growth, Repair, and Remineralization. Amsterdam: Elsevier Excerpta Medica-North Holland, 1973:169–182.

3. Burwell RG. Osteogenesis in cancellous bone grafts: Considered in terms of cellular changes, basic mechanisms in the perspective of growth control, and possible aberrations. Clin Orthop Related Res 1965;40: 35–47.

4. Burwell RG. Studies in transplantation of bone. J Bone Joint Surg 1960;B,48:432–566.

5. Boyne PJ. Induction of bone repair of various bone graft materials. In: Sognnaes RF (ed). Proceedings of the CIBA Foundation Symposium No. 11 on Hard Tissue Growth, Repair, and Remineralization. Amsterdam: Elsevier Excerpta Medica-North Holland, 1973: 121–141.

Chapter 2

Bone Grafts: Mechanisms

The use of bone grafts involves three mechanisms: *conduction*, *induction*, and *guided tissue regeneration*, which formerly was termed osteophylic response. All are involved in bone regeneration.

Bone Conduction

Conduction involves the use of inert bone substitute materials or nonviable autogenous and allogeneic banked bone grafts, which offer little or no inductive stimulation to the pluripotential cells of the host defect but do serve as scaffolding over which the bone-forming cells of the host may grow (Fig 2-1a). Particulate conductive materials can be placed, for example, between the root-form implant and the tooth extraction socket wall so that the bone repair can more rapidly proceed from the socket wall to the implanted surface, stimulating bone formation and integration of the root-form implant. Thus, conduction is used mostly in those defects in which there are three bony walls and in surgical sites in which a good supply of osteoblastic cells is provided by the bony walls (Fig 2-1b).

Conductive materials alone should not be used on single bony surfaces, such as the crest of the alveolar ridge, in an effort to encourage bone to grow outwardly from that bone interface. In this situation, the supply of osteoblasts available is not sufficient to produce the osteogenesis necessary to regenerate bone on the surface of the edentulous alveolar ridge; therefore, a highly inductive bone graft material that supplies the pluripotential cells necessary to regenerate the area should be used. Thus, for example, an iliac-crest bone graft with cancellous bone and high inductive capacities should be used to regenerate the ridge height of large edentulous areas. (We have been able to produce minimal new bone formation on cortical ridge surfaces in dogs, but only after perforation of the host bone cortex with a bur to open the underlying marrow-vascular spaces having an appropriate supply of osteogenic cells, and only after maintaining a supracortical space by means of a metal chamber. The amount of supracortical bone produced by bone conductor materials alone using this technique is not clinically significant. Therefore it is felt that inductive autograft material, in conjunction with conductive material, should be considered a necessary part of such grafting procedures.[1])

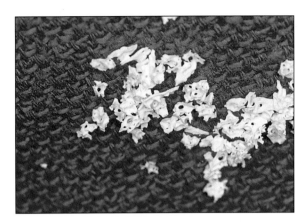

Fig 2-1a Natural porous bone mineral (Bio-Oss, Geistlich Sons/Osteohealth Co) showing high porosity and increased surface area, which is available for conduction.

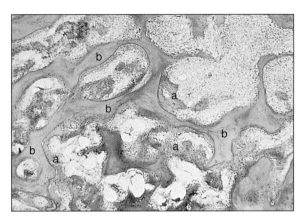

Fig 2-1b Center of a three-walled defect in which a cancellous bone mineral graft has been placed. New bone of the host (a) is growing over the latticework of a porous bone mineral graft (b), which is offering surfaces to enhance the ability of the defect to regenerate itself. Such bone-conductive grafts work well in two- or three-walled defects. These types of graft are not indicated for the surface of the alveolar ridge, where only one bony wall of the host is available to revascularize the graft particles.

If bone grafts are used in children for cleft palate repair, the growth of the child and the large numbers of pluripotential cells available in the growing child's bony surfaces are conducive to "induction" of the bone graft material, and to a favorable result. Thus, the bony recipient site itself can be "inductive." Clinicians are conditioned to think that it is necessary to add something to the bone graft (eg, exogenous growth factor materials) to produce the inductive effects. However, the recipient site itself may serve as an inductor of the bone-reparative cells[2] (Fig 2-2).

Conductive materials are used in three major areas of clinical concern (Fig 2-3):

1. In two- or three-walled bony defects with ample supply of pluripotential cells
2. As a carrier for bone inductors, eg, as a substrate for rhBMP-2 that releases the inductor over an appropriate period of time (Fig 2-4)
3. To increase bone density and to produce slow remodeling in the area. This remodeling ensures both the prolonged presence of bone mineral and a thickened trabecular pattern for a protective response to the occlusal and functional changes that may occur in the lifetime of the root-form implant.

Bone Induction

Bone Morphogenetic Protein (BMP)

One of the bone growth factor materials that can bring about induction of bone in areas in which bone regeneration would not normally occur (eg, the crest of the ridge of the maxilla) is rhBMP-2. This material can be obtained in a highly refined form by genetic engineering

Fig 2-2 Inductive responses, in which the bone graft induces its own pluripotential cells to become osteoblasts. The graft is also affecting the host defect itself, which has pluripotential cells that may be available in the defect wall and that may contribute to the bone regeneration by forming osteoblasts through the same inductive process.

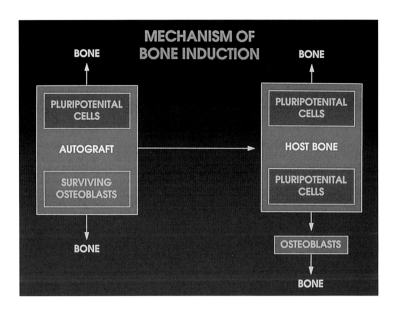

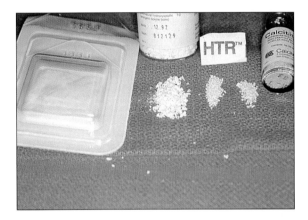

Fig 2-3 Possible carriers for rhBMP: (left to right) collagen sponge, porous bone mineral (Bio-Oss), polyhydroxyethyl methacrylate (PHEMA) spheres (HTR [hard-tissue replacement]; Bioplant, Inc, New York, NY), and hydroxyapatite particles.

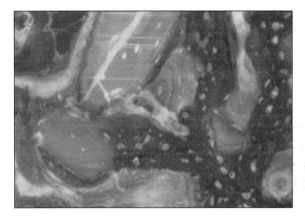

Fig 2-4 Effect of slowly remodeling Bio-Oss particles, which are carriers for BMP-2. The thickness of trabeculae of newly formed bone is increased surrounding particles of Bio-Oss (center left), which contain rhBMP-2. Photomicrograph taken at 4 weeks from a femoral defect of a rhesus monkey. (Original magnification ×120.)

using recombinant DNA.[3] This growth factor, when used in a surgically appropriate manner, is able to stimulate the pluripotential or precursor cells of the existing host wall and even the pluripotential cells in the cancellous portion of any bone graft that may be placed along with the inductor material.

In addition, rhBMP-2 may be simply placed on a carrier without any concomitant use of autogenous cancellous bone at the time.[4,5] Regeneration of large critical sized discontinuity defects by use of rhBMP-2 in a simple collagen sponge has been demonstrated[5] (Figs 2-5a to 2-5d). Such restored hemimandibulectomy

Bone Grafts: Mechanisms

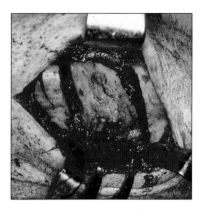

Fig 2-5a Hemimandibulectomy in a mature rhesus monkey, leaving a defect of approximately 2.2 cm in length.

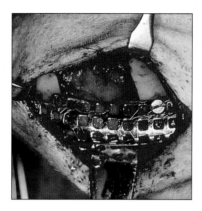

Fig 2-5b Discontinuity defect being maintained in a distended position by the use of titanium mesh. The area is not bone grafted but is merely implanted with a collagen sponge impregnated with rhBMP-2.

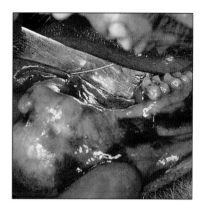

Fig 2-5c Regeneration of the area 3 months postoperatively.

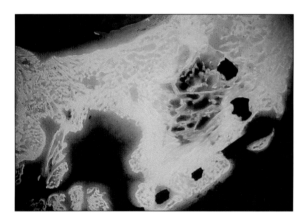

Fig 2-5d Fluorescence microscopic view of the regenerated area, showing excellent reformation of bone bridging the large discontinuity defect. Tetracycline-induced fluorescence indicates bone formation during the third postoperative month. There is a concentration of bone repair at the crest of the new alveolar ridge in the defect area (original magnification ×10).

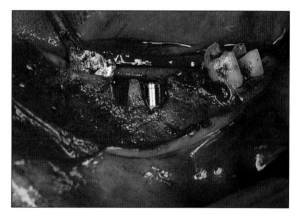

Fig 2-5e Steri-Oss implants (Steri-Oss, Inc, Yorba Linda, CA) placed in the BMP-regenerated mandibular defect. The reconstructed bone has excellent remodeling; new cortex has been formed.

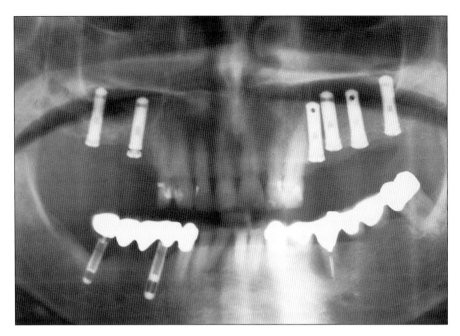

Fig 2-6 Patient with Steri-Oss implants on the left side that have been placed in antral bone formed by previous placement of rhBMP-2. On the right, two implants have been placed in an antral floor reconstructed with a particulate marrow and cancellous bone graft (PMCB) and Bio-Oss. The two methods of bone regeneration are being compared by clinical and radiographic examination.

defects in Macaca fascicularis have been shown to support root-form implants in full function for 6 to 8 months (Fig 2-5e). Bone morphogenetic protein–induced bone in the antral floor of patients also has supported implants for prostheses (Fig 2-6).

Demineralized Freeze-dried Bone

In the past, demineralized freeze-dried bone has been used by some surgeons on the premise that it is an "inductive material." However, there is very little inductive capacity in demineralized freeze-dried bone, because there is very little BMP in the product. Therefore, the effect of demineralized bone powder is primarily one of conduction and not induction. This material should not be used in an effort to build bone superiorly on the crest of the ridge of the maxilla or the mandible, unless it is used in conjunction with the autogenous bone grafts of the type previously described or as a carrier for true BMP in the concentrated, recombinant-DNA–produced biologic form (rhBMP).

Carriers for Inductive Substances

The growth factor rhBMP-2 is both a mitogen and a morphogen, and its functions are both to recruit progenitor cells and to morphologically change cells to the osteoblastic line of cellular maturation to produce bone. Such an effect may be needed for a short or long period, depending on the defect being regenerated. Carrier materials for rhBMP can be designed for a short-term, a medium-term, or a long-term effect, depending on the desired time of release of the rhBMP in the regenerating area.

Examples of materials that will carry rhBMP and be degraded over a short period (2 to 4 weeks) are collagen sponge and various degradable alloplastic materials (eg, polylactic acid and polyglycolic acid). Carriers that will release rhBMP over a slightly longer period are more slowly degradable. This class of materials would include such substances as calcium carbonate and tricalcium phosphate. Carriers that will release rhBMP over a long period are those that are slowly remodeled and resorbed, such as porous bone mineral (Bio-Oss; for a complete discussion, see the Appendix, "Characterization of Xenogeneic Bone Mineral," by Michael Peetz). Examples of carriers that are relatively inert and degraded very slightly, or not at all, are HTR (hard tissue replacement), which is a polyhydroxyethyl methacrylate (PHEMA) product in the form of beads, and certain types of porous hydroxyapatite.

Thus, a significant part of the clinical effect of the use of rhBMP may be determined by the degradability and other characteristics of the carrier itself. It is believed that the best type of carrier for rhBMP surrounding a root-form titanium implant may be a material that is slowly degradable, providing prolonged bone induction and availability for remodeling to obtain a higher density of cancellous bone resistant to future bone resorptive processes.[6]

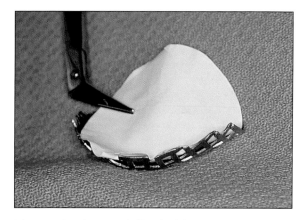

Fig 2-7 Titanium mesh lined with a membrane material with a pore size of 0.5 μm.

Osteophylic Response or Guided Tissue Regeneration

Exclusion of Cells

The term *guided tissue regeneration* is now used to describe the phenomenon in which alloplastic membrane surfaces exclude various types of cells from a surgical defect site. This phenomenon, formerly called osteophylic response,[7-9] was used extensively by us, beginning in 1965, in connection with bone grafting of large trauma-induced, and postoncologic defects.

The effect of the membrane depends on its pore size. If the pores are large, many of the cells (including fibroblasts) that the surgeon usually wishes to exclude will migrate through, allowing soft tissue, instead of new osseous matrix, to form in the bony defect. Normally a membrane with pores on the order of 0.5 μm is used; one with pores of 100.0 μm or more would allow a great many unwanted cells to enter the regenerating defect area (Fig 2-7).

Appropriate Use of Barrier Membranes

Whether a membrane-type barrier should be used in bone grafting for regeneration of the maxilla, for example, depends on the type of prosthetic restoration to be used. If the area is to be restored with a removable prosthesis requiring a deep vestibule for retention, a membrane should not be used because membranes tend to prevent a new periosteum from forming underneath the titanium next to the generating bone. Without the new periosteum, it is not possible to reposition the oral mucosa by suturing the mucosal flap at a superior level to reconstruct the vestibule after the removal of the titanium mesh.

If a membrane is not used with the titanium mesh, a new periosteal surface forms beneath the metal and overlying the regenerating bone. This newly formed periosteum will be thick and nonfriable and will retain the sutures used to attach the mucosa to produce an excellent vestibular height when the metal mesh is removed after 3 to 5 months. This vestibule-producing technique is really a secondary epithelialization procedure.

If the surgeon and the prosthodontist are restoring the area with root-form implants and a fixed prosthesis, a deep vestibule is of lesser importance. If root-form implants are being used, a membrane may be placed inside the titanium mesh and the mucosa merely closed over to the crest of the ridge following the removal of the mesh. The optimal effect of the membrane is to exclude the ingrowth of fibrous tissue, thereby increasing bone formation. However, if the use of the membrane would prevent the surgical development of a desirable vestibule, then the membrane should not be used.

Membranes should not be used when there are insufficient bony walls to provide the critical mass of precursor cells necessary to form bone. If the surgical defect has only one bony wall with very few cells available for osseous regeneration, the effect of the membrane would be to exclude the pluripotential precursor cells from the *periosteal flap*, thus excluding the necessary additional pool of cells that would be available if the membrane were not used. Therefore, the filter or membrane should not be used when there is only one bony wall with a poor blood supply that offers a diminished number of cells to regenerate the defect.[1]

If, however, the defect has a minimum of three bony walls with excellent vascularity and a good reservoir of pluripotential cells from the host bone available to be induced to form osteoblasts and bone, the membrane may be used. The cells from the periosteum can be excluded, because they will not be necessary for appropriate regeneration of the defect. An excellent example of a complete, functional, and anatomically correct reconstruction of a large defect by using the membrane system is shown in Figs 2-8a to 2-8c.[8,9] When cells from the mucoperiosteal flap are excluded, a large amount of fibrous tissue will be prevented from entering the bone-regenerating area; this effect will contribute to an excellent result when used in an appropriate surgical bone site (Figs 2-8 and 2-9).

For enhancement of bone density in the final reconstructive product, a 50-50 mixture of PMCB with Bio-Oss has been found to be most effective[10,11] (Fig 2-10).

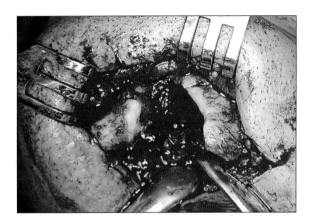

Fig 2-8a Defect of the mandible in a Vietnam War casualty with a large fragment of missing symphyseal bone, a discontinuity defect, and a comminuted fracture of the mandible resulting from a mortar-induced injury.

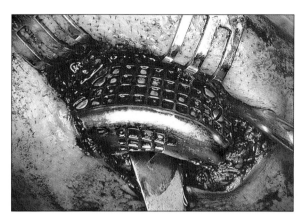

Fig 2-8b Area of the inferior border of the mandible grafted by PMCB in a chrome-cobalt mesh.

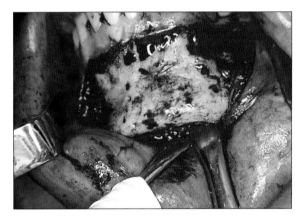

Fig 2-8c Resulting reconstruction after removal of the chrome-cobalt mesh 6 months after grafting. The effect of the metal mesh in dictating the contour of the regeneration, the inductive effect of the PMCB graft in the host bone site, and the use of the membrane to prevent the intrusion of fibrous tissue in the area all have combined to promote the high quality of regeneration that has occurred.

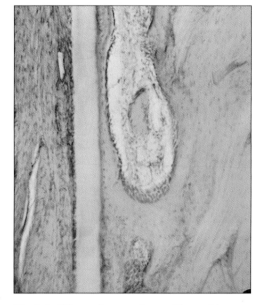

Fig 2-9 Effect of a membrane filter with a pore size of less than 1.0 µm. The membrane has excluded all the fibrous tissue, which remains on the outside (left) of the white line (the membrane). On the inside of the defect (right), bone is forming against the membrane's surface without intrusion of any fibrous tissue in the healing area (original magnification ×50).

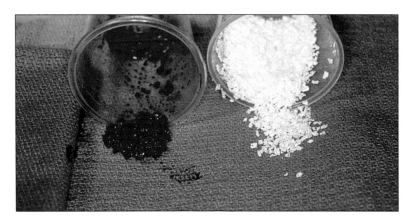

Fig 2-10 Appropriate mixture of porous bone mineral (Bio-Oss) with particulate autogenous cancellous bone. This is the optimal particle size of the PMCB.

References

1. Richter HE, Surg WE, Boyne PJ. Stimulation of osteogenesis in the dog mandible by autogenous bone marrow transplants. Oral Surg, Oral Med, and Oral Path 1968;26(3):396–405.

2. Boyne PJ. Maxillofacial surgery. In Habal M (ed). Bone Grafts and Bone Substitutes. Philadelphia: Saunders, 1992:291–298.

3. Wozney JM, Rosen V, Celeste AJ, Mitsock LM, Whitters MJ, Kriz RW, Hewick RM, Wang EA. Novel regulators of bone formation: Molecular clones and activities. Science 1988;242:1528–1534.

4. Riedel GE. Clinical and preclinical studies with rhBMP-2. In: Hollinger J (ed). Proceedings of the Portland Bone Symposium. Portland: Oregon Health Sciences University, 1995:597–601.

5. Boyne PJ. Animal studies of application of rhBMP-2 in maxillofacial reconstruction. In: Hollinger J (ed). Proceedings of the Portland Bone Symposium. Portland: Oregon Health Sciences University, 1995:602–617.

6. Boyne PJ, Urist M. Evaluation of bone mineral carriers for bone morphogenetic protein. In: Boyne PJ (ed). Proceedings of the 4th International Congress in Preprosthetic Surgery. Palm Springs, CA, Apr 18–20, 1991.

7. Boyne PJ. Regeneration of alveolar bone beneath cellulose acetate filter implants. J Dent Res 1964;43:827.

8. Boyne PJ. Tissue transplantation. In: Kruger GO (ed). Oral and Maxillofacial Surgery, ed 5. St Louis: Mosby, 1979:196–198, 283–286, 296, 298.

9. Boyne PJ. Restoration of osseous defects in maxillofacial casualties. J Am Dent Assoc 1969;78:767–776.

10. Boyne PJ. Use of porous bone mineral to increase bone density. In: Proceedings of Materials Research Society Fall 1993 Symposium, Boston. Material Research Proceedings 1993;331:263–268.

11. Boyne PJ. Vergleich von Bio-Oss und anderen Implantationsmaterialien bei der Erhaltung des Alveolarkammes des Unterkiefers beim Menschen. Unfallheilkunde 1991;216:98–103.

Part II

Surgical Reconstruction Using Titanium Mesh in Combination with Bone Grafts

Chapter 3

For Restoration with Conventional Prostheses

Biocompatibility of Titanium Mesh

Physical Properties

The physical properties of titanium metal that relate to effectiveness in surgical practice are principally those that affect fatigue strength, corrosion in bodily fluids, surface cleanliness, and malleability.

Fatigue Strength

In general, pure titanium material does not undergo corrosion in the mammalian body. However, its fatigue strength can be affected by a number of factors. RL Skaggs of the University of Nevada compared the fatigue resistance of titanium maxillofacial mesh material (TiMesh; TiMesh, Inc, Las Vegas, NV) with other types of titanium product (unpublished data, 1993). The TiMesh product exhibited longer fatigue life than did other processed and commercially available titanium materials that were tested. TiMesh produced a fatigue test result of 6,500,000 cycles, whereas other types of titanium material failed at 350,000 to 450,000 cycles, indicating that TiMesh is far superior.

Purity

The purity of the TiMesh surface also has been evaluated. It was shown that the surface of this titanium metal is uncontaminated with any other type of metallic debris. Common contaminants such as chloride, silicon, calcium, and iron were found on the surfaces of other titanium products, but not on the TiMesh material. Scanning electron microscopy has been used to evaluate the titanium oxide surface on the metal product. Such a coating is not regarded as a contaminant but rather as a desired metal passivated surface. A metal is defined as clean from a surgical implant standpoint if the characteristics of the mass of the material are demonstrable completely to the periphery without a change of chemical composition and no foreign species are detected.[1] Skaggs has reported (unpublished data, 1993) that the TiMesh material has a metallic composition that does extend from the bulk of the material to the surface.

In addition, the method of preparation of the mesh and the rounded corners of TiMesh tend to produce a smooth surface that is free of contamination. Figure 3-1a shows the rounded corners of the material, which is produced by a process designed to decrease the amount of

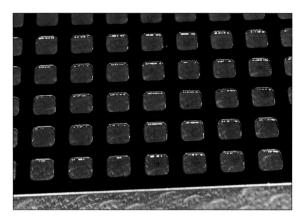

Fig 3-1a TiMesh. The surface of the square mesh is slightly rounded.

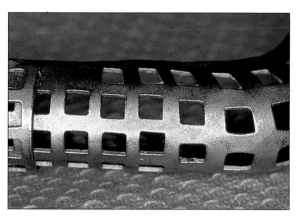

Fig 3-1b Another type of titanium mesh. The squares are sharply cut and have rough edges.

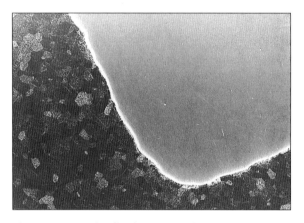

Fig 3-2a Longitudinal cross-sectional photomicrograph of TiMesh, the corner of the mesh hole is rounded. (Original magnification ×50.) Note the smooth, contaminant-free surface of a normal, continuous surface to bulk, titanium microstructure. (Courtesy of R. L. Skaggs, TiMesh)

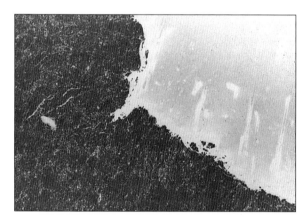

Fig 3-2b Longitudinal cross-sectional photomicrograph of another type of titanium mesh produced by a different method and another manufacturer. The edge of the mesh hole is sharp. (Original magnification ×50.) Note the roughened surface, indicating an abnormal titanium microstructure. (Courtesy of R. L. Skaggs, TiMesh)

fatigue fracture and contamination. Another type of titanium mesh has sharp edges (Fig 3-1b). Figures 3-2a and 3-2b show the TiMesh surface and the surface of another titanium mesh product. Note the sharp edges of the other mesh and the rounded corners of the TiMesh.

Ductility and Tensile Strength

Other properties of titanium mesh that have been investigated include hardness, tensile strength, and ductility (Skaggs RL, unpublished data, 1993). These evaluations have shown that some other types of titanium have very

Biocompatibility of Titanium Mesh

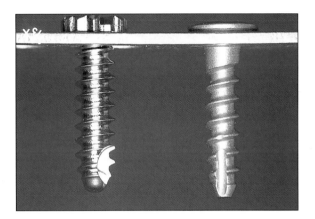

Fig 3-3a TiMesh screw (left), showing the true configuration of a self-tapping, self-threading surface. The groove configuration near the tip accommodates bone as it is cut from the osteotomy site by the screw. This modification allows the excess bone to come to the surface as the screw is placed. The non–self-tapping screw (right) does not have this configuration. Such a screw, as it is driven to place, will tend to compress the wall of the osteotomy hole, leading to bone necrosis, a decrease in pullout resistance, and a tendency for the screw to loosen with time.

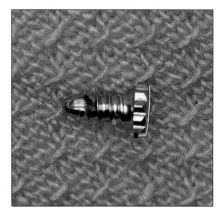

Fig 3-3b Small self-tapping screw with the same configuration near the tip to relieve compression against the walls of the screw hole as the screw is placed.

low ductility and flexibility. Such plates must be made thicker, of necessity, to impart the strength necessary to contain grafts and to contain the host bone fragments in maxillofacial surgery. TiMesh has excellent properties of ductility and flexibility, so that the material can be made thinner with very little possibility of fracture. The less rigid plates of TiMesh also have a very high tensile strength, which permits microfluctuation of the host bone when stressed. Thus, stress shielding of the bone by the titanium mesh implant is minimal or nonexistent. It is apparent that other, heavier orthopedic plates do have the possibility of producing stress shielding and as such may diminish the full potential of bone repair and remodeling of bone grafts (Skaggs RL, unpublished data, 1993; Morgan F, personal communication, 1996).

Self-tapping Screws

The pure titanium mesh utilized in this study is made to be held in place by commercially pure titanium self-tapping screws. Self-tapping screws are designed to be placed after preparation of an unthreaded, or untapped, pilot hole with an appropriately sized bur. Self-tapping, self-threading screws can be identified by an open portion near the distal end of the screw designed to accommodate shavings of bone, which are removed from the margins of the osseous hole as the threaded portion of the titanium screws are placed (Figs 3-3a and 3-3b). As the screw is placed, the shaved bone particles are delivered by the screw threads to the surface of the bone under the head of the screw. Non–self-tapping screws do not perform in this manner and a pre-tapped threaded hole

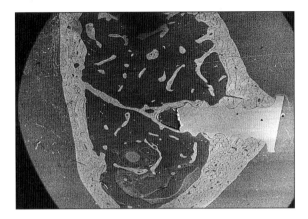 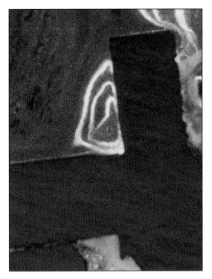

Fig 3-4a Macroscopic view of a TiMesh screw in place in the mandible of a monkey. The trabecular pattern is concentrated and increased in density near the tip of the screw, and lamellated bone is increased near the screw neck extending to the head of the screw. The surface of the screw is well-integrated, one of the reasons for the high strength and pullout resistance of this screw design.

Fig 3-4b Cross section of titanium mesh at the cortical surface of the mandible in a rhesus monkey. The mesh has been in place for 15 months. The tetracycline label was administered at 1-month intervals, at 12, 13, and 14 months. The fluorescence label reveals an increase in lamellated bone on the surface around the titanium mesh, indicating a permanency of the integration of the bone with the metal. This leads to excellent configuration of the mesh when used in the treatment of fractures and in the treatment of large bony lesions with bone grafts. The mesh in these cases may remain in place permanently, covered by the well-lamellated and mature remodeled bone.

must be prepared in the bone. Pressure against the sides of the screw hole by non–self-threading instruments can cause interfacial resorption of bone and loosening of the screw postoperatively.

Work reported by Boyle et al[2] has demonstrated that the self-tapping screws of the TiMesh system exhibit superior pullout strength and have less possibility of stripping the bone than do other commonly used chrome, cobalt, titanium alloy, or commercially pure titanium self-tapping screws. The same parameters were used to show that the TiMesh screws are superior to non–self-tapping types. The 2.2-mm TiMesh self-tapping screw produces the largest stripping torque, the largest numerical difference between insertion and stripping torques, and the greatest pullout strength of all the screws tested.[2] This study indicated the superiority of the TiMesh fixation device in the placement of titanium mesh sheets containing bone grafts for reconstruction of large bony defects as well as in the fixation of fractured facial bones.

Our work has shown (PJB, unpublished data) that both the TiMesh self-tapping screws and the TiMesh materials integrate well with host bone, allowing progressive osseous remodeling and formation of lamellated bone with the passage of time and the final effect of long-term function (Figs 3-4a and 3-4b).

Advantages of TiMesh Materials

In addition to the high ductility, high strength, and purity of the surface of the product, the method of preparation and perforation of the squares of the TiMesh material prevents titanium fractures and the propagation of microfractures. Ordinary titanium mesh that is manufactured by other means has the tendency to fracture at the angles of the square openings of the mesh.

The configuration of the TiMesh self-tapping screws is superior. In addition, the mesh plate has high purity and has physical properties that are close to those of cortical bone. Furthermore, the metal mesh does not produce stress shielding. All these qualities are very much desired in a product of this type to promote the probability of surgical success.

Surgical Maxillary Reconstruction

The combined use of titanium mesh and grafting of particulate marrow and cancellous bone (PMCB) has been employed for the past 25 years in the reconstruction of varying degrees of bone deficiencies in atrophic maxillas.[3] The technique employs one of two thicknesses of titanium mesh (either 0.020 or 0.015 inch) in which the "land area" of the mesh is designed to present approximately 4-mm openings.[3] These thicknesses and this degree of opening are ideal for the reconstruction of the deficient anterior maxilla or for the restoration of a totally missing maxillary alveolar ridge resulting from marked generalized atrophic changes from tuberosity to tuberosity. The titanium mesh maintains an appropriate contour for the desired osseous restoration of the maxilla and supplies the proper submucosal support of the bone graft to withstand modified occlusal function during the time the titanium mesh is in place (usually 3 to 6 months). Following the removal of the titanium mesh, a secondary epithelialization surgical procedure is performed to create a vestibule.

The surgical technique for reconstruction of the osseous base of the deficient atrophic maxilla to allow conventional prosthodontic replacement will be described in the remainder of this chapter.

Presurgical Procedures

A supramucosal alginate impression of the deficient maxilla is made. A stone or plaster cast is poured and waxed up in the area where the bone regeneration is desired (Figs 3-5a and 3-5b). This waxed-up cast is then duplicated in acrylic resin and the acrylic resin cast is used as a template base for swedging of the titanium mesh, which is taken from a flat stock of approximately 4 x 8-inch titanium. The mesh is either 0.015 or 0.020 inch thick. A piece of baseplate wax is placed over the cast in the area of the desired bony reconstruction (Fig 3-6). The baseplate wax is then taken from the cast and flattened against the flat stock of titanium, and the mesh is cut out on the bias (Fig 3-7).

The resulting cut-out of mesh is then swedged to the acrylic resin cast (Fig 3-8a). In the swedging procedure, a temporary screw is placed in the midline of the palatal portion of the acrylic resin cast to maintain the mesh in place during swedging process. The palatal portion of the mesh is cut out as an extension on the midline of the palate to accept one or two screws in the exact midline symphysis of the palatal bone (Fig 3-8b). The palatal suture area is thicker and will accept approximately 7- to 9-mm-long screws, which will usually be sufficient to maintain the mesh and the graft in place.

For Restoration with Conventional Prostheses

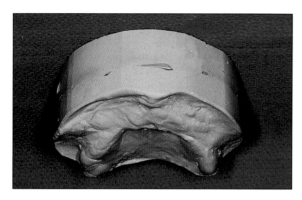

Fig 3-5a Cast of a completely edentulous maxilla with anterior deficiency.

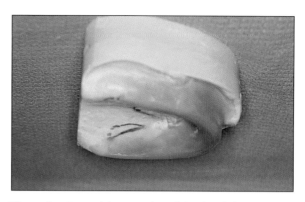

Fig 3-5b Cast with wax placed in the defect area to build the maxilla to the desired size and shape. This cast will be duplicated in acrylic resin.

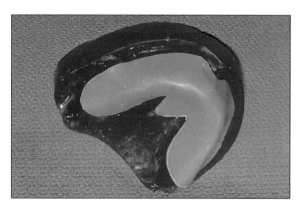

Fig 3-6 Baseplate wax placed over the acrylic resin cast in the area of the desired restoration to form a pattern for the titanium mesh.

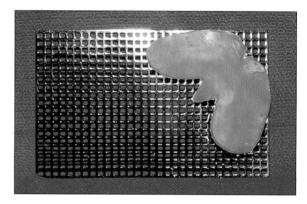

Fig 3-7 Baseplate wax flattened against the flat titanium mesh to form a pattern to cut the mesh. The mesh is cut out on the bias around the pattern and adapted to the cast.

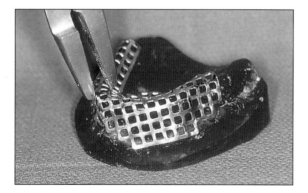

Fig 3-8a Swedging of the titanium mesh to the cast with special pliers.

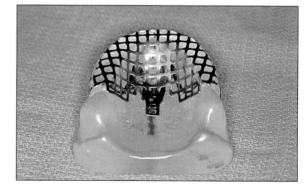

Fig 3-8b Titanium mesh adapted to the cast. A palatal mesh extension is present to accommodate a 7-mm-long screw to secure the mesh and graft in place.

Surgical Maxillary Reconstruction

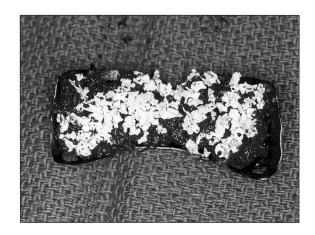

Fig 3-9 Titanium mesh with the porous bone mineral and the PMCB graft. The porous bone mineral is mixed in a 50-50 proportion in the center portion of the graft. The peripheral portion directly underneath the titanium mesh is entirely PMCB autograft. Porous bone mineral alone is placed immediately next to the host bone.

All the rough edges of the metal are then cut and smoothed with a diamond bur or carborundum wheel. The entire mesh is cleaned and sterilized by autoclaving.

Placement of Titanium Mesh and Graft Material

For graft placement, the deficient bone site is exposed by making a mid-crestal incision from tuberosity to tuberosity without using anterior vertical releasing incisions. The mucoperiosteum is elevated as one complete flap and the bony ridge is exposed. If necessary, a slight diagonal, vertical incision may be made extending posteriorly from the tuberosities. At the time of surgery, the mesh is filled with the particulate bone graft material, which is usually composed of autogenous cancellous bone that is cut to particle sizes of approximately 2 mm in diameter.[1]

During the past 8 years, we have been adding bovine porous bone mineral (Bio-Oss, Geistlich Sons/Osteohealth Co) to the particulate autograft. This material is added in approximately a 50-50 mixture by volume (Fig 3-9). The conductive porous bone mineral is used to increase bone density. The clinical effect of this increase in restored bone density will be discussed later in this book.

When the graft material is placed in the contained titanium mesh, care is taken not to place the porous bone mineral immediately beneath the titanium metal. A layer of autogenous cancellous bone alone is always placed in this area. The reason for this placement and layering of the graft material is to have an autogenous cellular substrate located immediately beneath the titanium mesh in the event of a dehiscence so that the dehisced area will expose viable cells of the autograft and not the nonviable Bio-Oss (Figs 3-9 and 3-10). Particulate autogenous marrow and cancellous bone is able to withstand the insult of dehiscence, whereas cortical autogenous bone particles, other conductive allogeneic materials, and porous bone xenogeneic mineral particles when used alone are not able to withstand the exposure and the insult of exposure to the environment of the oral cavity.

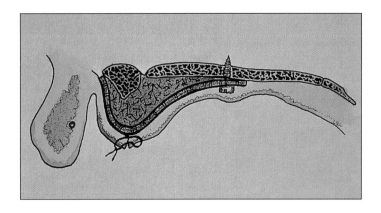

Fig 3-10 Placement of the titanium mesh and PMCB graft for an anterior maxillary deficiency. The mesh and graft are held by a single midline screw placed in the palatal symphysis.

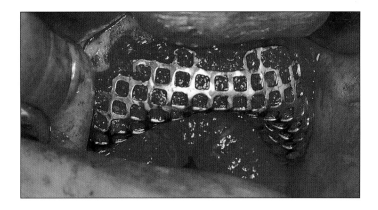

Fig 3-11 Placement of particulate graft material, composed of PMCB, within titanium mesh over a maxillary defect. A bur hole has been placed and the mesh has been secured in place with a midpalatal screw. The exposure is obtained by means of an envelope soft-tissue flap without the use of vertical relaxing incisions.

Therefore, if the graft has been properly placed, dehiscence of the graft and metal is not cause for early removal of the metal mesh. If a dehiscence occurs postoperatively, the area is merely irrigated, and the titanium and the graft are allowed to remain in place for the planned 3- to 6-month interval.

The graft material is placed in the titanium mesh in layers. A layer of Bio-Oss is first placed next to the residual host ridge. This layer is followed by a 50-50 mixture of Bio-Oss and cancellous autogenous bone marrow (see Figs 3-9 and 3-10). The most inferior or peripheral portion of the graft, next to the titanium, is composed of a layer of autogenous cancellous bone and marrow used alone.

The mesh is then placed over the deficient ridge and the midline is carefully aligned with the palatal bone. An appropriate bur hole is made to accept the self-tapping titanium mesh screw, which will hold the mesh and graft in place (Figs 3-10 and 3-11).

For anterior maxillary deficiencies, the mesh is usually removed in 3 months. For larger areas and entirely deficient maxillas, the mesh is removed in 4 to 5 months. In cases of hemimaxillectomies and even greater deficient areas resulting from trauma and from oncologic surgery, the graft and the titanium mesh are allowed to remain in place for 5 to 6 months before removal because of the more massive areas of reconstruction and necessary bone regeneration involved.

Removal of Titanium Mesh

The surgical technique for titanium mesh removal involves making a midcrestal incision over the restored ridge of the maxilla from tuberosity to tuberosity and relaxing incisions placed posteriorly in the mucobuccal fold bilaterally (Fig 3-12). No other relaxing incisions are made at this time, and the buccal and labial portions of the mucoperiosteum are elevated as a single envelope flap laterally and anteriorly to expose the underlying titanium metal in the same manner used for the surgical exposure for the insertion of the graft (see Fig 3-12).

A No. 69 right-angle beaver blade is used to facilitate the dissection of the fibrous tissue from the titanium mesh (Fig 3-13a and 3-13b). This dissection is carried supraperiosteally to the subalar area in order to leave a good periosteal thickness of tissue above the titanium mesh (Fig 3-14). This thickness of soft tissue is necessary to complete the secondary epithelialization procedure, which will produce the new vestibule after the titanium mesh is removed.

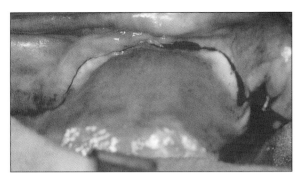

Fig 3-12 Incision for the removal of the titanium mesh and the graft. A midcrestal incision is made from tuberosity to tuberosity, exposing the underlying titanium mesh. A single buccal labial flap without relaxing excisions, except in the posterior tuberosity area, is raised. Anterior relaxing incisions tend to cause dehiscence; therefore, they are not usually made. The soft tissue is elevated, therefore, as one complete flap from the crest of the ridge.

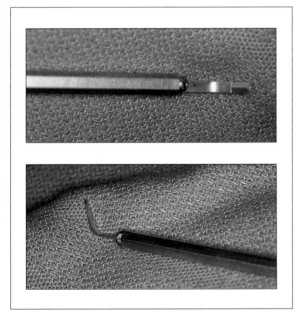

Figs 3-13a and 3-13b Two views of an angled beaver cleft palate scalpel, which is used to separate the connective tissue from the titanium mesh upon its removal. If a filter membrane has been used, this reflection is markedly facilitated. If the membrane has not been used, the beaver blade is employed to separate the tenacious fibrous tissue from the underlying new periosteum.

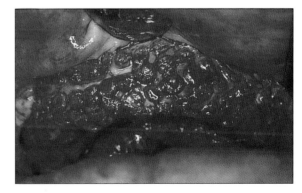

Fig 3-14 New, thick periosteal surface, seen after removal of the titanium mesh. The palatal mucosal flap is then sutured to the underlying new periosteum with chromic 3-0 and 4-0 interrupted sutures to create a new vestibule in a secondary epithelialization procedure.

For Restoration with Conventional Prostheses

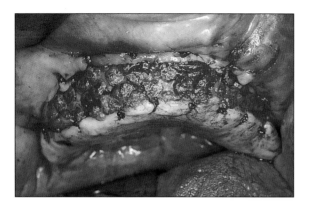

Fig 3-15 After completion of the vestibular-lengthening procedure at the time of removal of the titanium mesh, a portion of the new periosteum that varies from 8 to 14 mm in length remains. The denuded periosteal area will be completely re-epithelialized in 5 weeks.

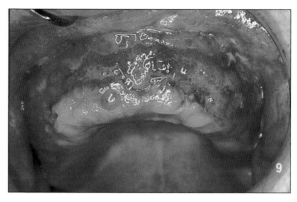

Fig 3-16 New epithelial surface that has formed in the area of the new exposed periosteum at the end of 6 weeks. The new epithelium has formed attached mucosa and will serve as an excellent soft-tissue surface and a base for a conventional prosthesis or, in the case of root-form implants, as an attached mucosal base (also see Figs 5-14d and 5-14e, which show re-epithelialization with root-form implants).

After exposure of the titanium mesh, the midpalatal titanium screws are removed and the titanium is gently elevated by grasping the posterior extent of the mesh with a heavy needle holder and bending the titanium toward the body of the titanium mesh itself. This maneuver prevents the tearing of the soft tissue and exposure of the underlying bone. As mentioned, it is necessary to keep the new soft tissue periosteum intact to complete the later vestibular-deepening procedure.

Creation of a Vestibule (Secondary Epithelialization Procedure)

When the soft tissue is closed after removal of the mesh, the palatal flap is first sutured to the underlying new periosteum at the crest of the ridge to secure the palatal mucosa and prevent formation of a hematoma. To create the new vestibule, the mucosal envelope flap that formerly was on the outside of the titanium is now sutured superiorly to the thickened new periosteum, which formerly was located beneath the titanium mesh between the mesh and the newly regenerated bone resulting from the grafting procedure. Chromic sutures, sizes 3-0 and 4-0, are used as a mattress stitch, picking up the underlying thick new periosteum and attaching the mucosal flap superiorly to produce the lengthened vestibule (Fig 3-15). After the vestibule has been created by this procedure, the area of exposed underlying new periosteum, which is not epithelialized and which is not covered with mucosa (ie, the area between the anterior labial extent of the palatal mucoperiosteal flap and the depth of the vestibule), is now approximately 8 to 14 mm in height (see Fig 3-15).

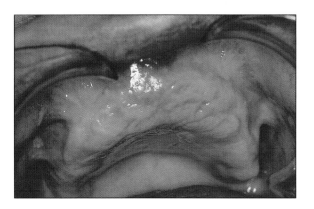

Fig 3-17a Ten-year postoperative view. A maxillary conventional complete denture has functioned well during that time. The PMCB graft has maintained alveolar height and width. Provided that there is excellent occlusal function and good balance of the occlusal forces, this bony area will be maintained under a maxillary conventional complete denture.

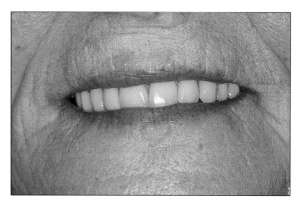

Fig 3-17b Conventional complete dentures in place over grafted maxillary ridge shown in Fig 3-17a.

A splint is then placed in the area to maintain the vestibular height during the secondary epithelialization period, which extends through the next 4 to 5 weeks postoperatively. At the end of 5 postoperative weeks, a new epithelial surface will have formed over the new exposed periosteal area; this area becomes attached mucosa (Fig 3-16). Excellent attached mucosa therefore forms against the alveolar ridge anteriorly and posteriorly, creating a vestibule for the conventional prosthesis. A definitive conventional prosthesis can be made at the end of the 5-week postoperative period, replacing the provisional prosthodontic replacement.

We have used this procedure for the past 25 years in the described manner utilizing autogenous bone grafts (Figs 3-17a and 3-17b). During the past 9 years, we have used the 50-50 graft mixture of porous bone mineral (Bio-Oss) and particulate autograft as described. (Prior to that time, we used an earlier porous bone mineral product developed by us in the Navy.[4,5] This material was also from a bovine source and was used in the manner described.) The material is subjected to an organic extraction process producing a product called "anorganic."[4,5]

In patients with good occlusion and properly balanced articulation, there is excellent restoration and preservation of the ridge. Ridge resorption is minimal over a 9- to 10-year period in our patients. We have followed approximately 50 patients over 9 years. The restored maxillas and mandibles have shown very little resorption[6] (only approximately 25% of the ridge height) over long postoperative observation periods, indicating the beneficial effect of the porous bone mineral in increasing bone density and decreasing resorption under conventional prostheses over a long period of function.

References

1. Kasemo B, Lausmaa J. Biomaterial and implant surfaces: On the role of cleanliness, contamination and preparation procedures. J Biomed Mater Res 1988; 22:145–158.

2. Boyle JM, Frost DE, Foley WL, Grady JJ. Torque and pullout analysis of six currently available self-tapping and "emergency" screws. J Oral Maxillofac Surg 1993;51:45–50.

3. Boyne PJ, Cole MD, Stringer DE, Shafquat JP. A technique for osseous restoration of deficient edentulous maxillary ridges. J Oral Maxillofac Surg 1985; 43:87–91.

4. Boyne PJ. The use of anorganic bone implants in oral surgery. J Oral Surg 1958;16:53–62.

5. Boyne PJ, Losee FL. Response of oral tissues to grafts of ethylene diamine treated heterogenous bone. [Research Report NM 004 006.09.02; Vol. 15: 283–310] Bethesda, MD: Navy Medical Research Institute, 1957.

6. Boyne PJ. Vergleich von Bio-Oss und anderen Implantationsmaterialien bei der Erhaltung des Alveolarkammes des Unterkiefers beim Menschen. Unfallheilkunde 1991;216:98–103.

Chapter 4

For Restoration With Root-Form Implants

Large Partially Edentulous Areas

In the reconstruction of partially edentulous areas that have bony defects due to old trauma or long-standing atrophy, it is necessary to reconstruct both the width and the height of the alveolar ridge. To generate the appropriate quantity of bone around root-form implants, it is necessary to reconstruct the maxilla both palatally and labially. When a conventional anterior prosthesis has been in function for many years, considerable loss of bone usually occurs in the subalar base area, as well as in the alveolar ridge itself, giving the face a flattened appearance and making the ridge an unesthetic and nonfunctional base for prosthetic restoration (Fig 4-1).

Placement of Titanium Mesh and Graft Material

The titanium mesh used for maxillary reconstruction with root-form implants is made with a technique similar to that employed for the complete conventional denture for an anterior deficiency. The stone cast is enhanced by waxing in the anterior area; care is taken to build the wax sufficiently labially and superiorly under the subalar base area.

In the case of an anticipated fixed prosthetic restoration or a fixed-removable replacement, it is necessary to have durable osseous reconstruction that will not resorb. In such cases, porous bone mineral (Bio-Oss, Geistlich Sons/Osteohealth Co) is utilized with the autogenous particulate marrow and cancellous bone (PMCB). As described in Chapter 3 (see Fig 3-9), the porous bone mineral is placed next to the host bony surface of the ridge and then intermixed with PMCB in layers built up to the occlusal surface area. The first layer over the existing bone base is, therefore, porous bone mineral. Autogenous graft material is used alone immediately beneath the titanium and beneath the mucosal surface as has been described for the reconstruction of the maxilla for a conventional prosthesis (Chapter 3).

When extreme atrophy has created a knife-edged ridge with a poor blood supply (Fig 4-2a and 4-2b), a nonresorbable filter membrane is not used, primarily because the periosteal blood supply and the pool of cells from the periosteal surface will be excluded from the re-

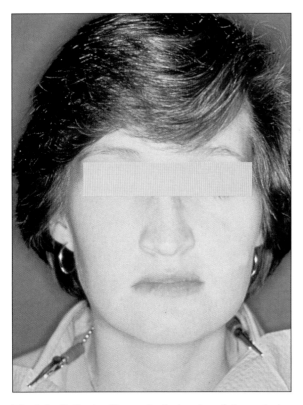

Fig 4-1 Patient with marked atrophy of the anterior maxilla in the area of previous trauma with loss of the premaxilla from canine to canine. The subalar base, is flattened and, esthetically, the maxilla appears deficient. (Treatment of this patient is shown in Figs 4-2 to 4-10.)

generating area if the membrane is used. Use of a membrane, therefore, would be counterproductive in effecting the anticipated restoration of the maxilla (Fig 4-3).

When the titanium mesh is used without a barrier membrane, the anterior extent of the maxilla may be reconstructed to a point 10 to 15 mm anterior to the anterior nasal spine. This anterior or labial reconstruction is shown in a comparison of preoperative and postoperative radiographs. The preoperative radiograph shows the deficient area, the preexisting fixed prosthesis, and a very small, knife-edged alveolar ridge. The preoperative prosthesis was supported only by soft tissue anterior to the anterior nasal spine (Fig 4-4a). The postoperative radiograph shows the extent to which the ridge has been effectively restored, some 12 mm anterior to the preoperative ridge (Fig 4-4b).

Removal of Titanium Mesh and Creation of a Vestibule

After the mix of porous bone mineral and particulate marrow and cancellous bone has been placed, a provisional prosthesis with modified

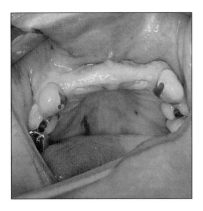

Fig 4-2a Atrophic, partially edentulous anterior maxilla.

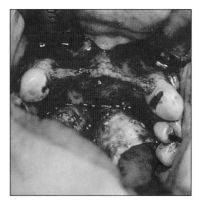

Fig 4-2b Severely knife-edged ridge of the deficient maxilla.

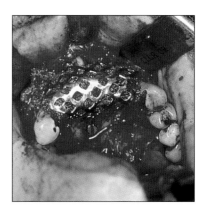

Fig 4-3 Titanium mesh in place over the partially edentulous area. The titanium mesh contains PMCB and porous bone mineral graft (Bio-Oss).

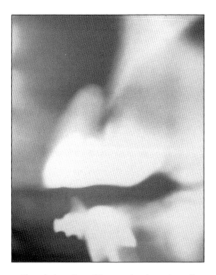
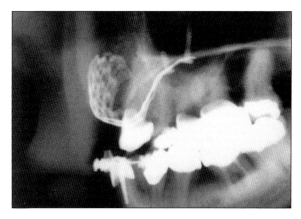

Fig 4-4a Preoperative lateral radiograph showing the preexisting fixed prosthesis situated anterior to the anterior nasal spine and anterior to the knife-edged ridge. The fixed prosthesis is suspended in soft tissue in an effort to create an esthetic appearance.

Fig 4-4b Postoperative view of the titanium mesh in place. The anterior portion of the maxillary ridge can be built to more than 12 mm anterior to the previous location of the anterior nasal spine.

function is used for 4 months. The titanium mesh is removed after 4 to 5 months. Thick new periosteum will be found overlying the alveolar ridge and a new cortex of bone will have been established (Figs 4-5a and 4-5b). This tissue establishes the basis for the proper restoration of the vestibule, in which the mucosal surface that formerly was overlying the titanium mesh is now sutured to the new periosteum, producing an excellent basis for secondary epithelialization and for the reformation of attached mucosa (Fig 4-6). The area of the secondary epithelialization is protected by a splint (Fig 4-7). Within 5 weeks, new attached mucosa will be established over the new periosteal surface.

Placement of Implants

At the time of removal of the titanium mesh, root-form implants are placed in the new bony ridge. The thick reformed new periosteal surface is used as a soft-tissue covering over the sealing screws of the implants (Fig 4-8). The implants are allowed to integrate for 4 to 5 months before they are uncovered (Fig 4-9). Through this technique, a marked improvement in facial contour and in the subalar base can be achieved (Fig 4-10).

Root-form implants also may be placed simultaneously with the titanium mesh and the Bio-Oss particulate autogenous graft mixture if there is sufficient residual host bone to stabilize the implants at the time of placement (Fig 4-11). This stabilization will require approximately 5 mm of bone height on the crest of the ridge. The remainder of the root-form implant surface can interface with the bone graft material. The resultant osseous integration of the titanium surface will then involve approximately 4 to 5 mm of residual host bone, and the remainder of the 10 to 12 mm of the implant length will achieve integration from the maturation and remodeling of the graft itself.

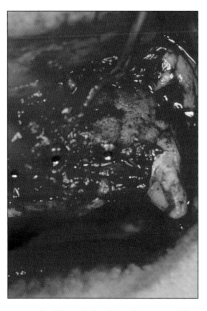
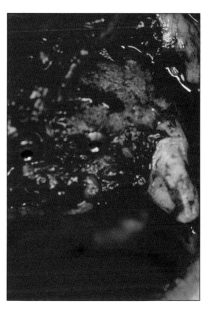

Fig 4-5a Reconstructed ridge (left side of premaxilla) at the time of removal of the titanium mesh, 4 months postoperatively. An excellent bony base and a thick new periosteal layer have been established. This periosteal layer will serve as a base for a new attached mucosa in a secondary epithelialization procedure.

Fig 4-5b Underlying bony regenerated cortex. A new bone cortex has formed, some 12 mm anterior to the previous crest of the alveolar ridge. The periosteum has been excised in this case only to demonstrate the underlying cortical bone. Normally, the new periosteum would not be disturbed and would be used as the basis for increasing the vestibular depth in the secondary epithelialization procedure.

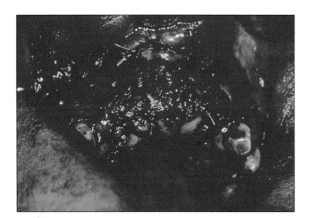
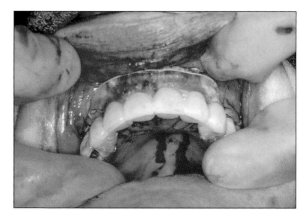

Fig 4-6 Mucosa sutured to the depth of the vestibule. The flap is attached to the thick new periosteum, establishing a new vestibule.

Fig 4-7 Splint placed following the secondary epithelialization procedure and placement of the root-form implants.

Fig 4-8 Root-form implants placed at the time of removal of the titanium mesh. The thick new periosteum is used as a soft-tissue covering over the implants. A new mucosal surface is not needed at this time, because secondary epithelialization of the area will occur in 5 weeks.

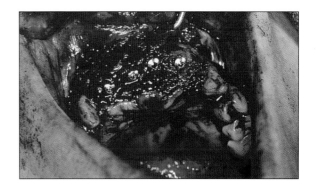

Fig 4-9 Uncovering of the implants. New attached mucosa is seen in the area of the secondary epithelialization procedure, establishing excellent vestibular height. This epithelialization is complete within 5 weeks of the establishing of the new vestibular height. (Compare with Fig 4-2b.)

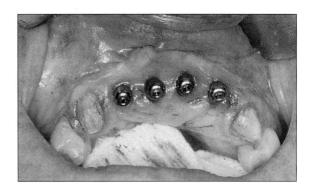

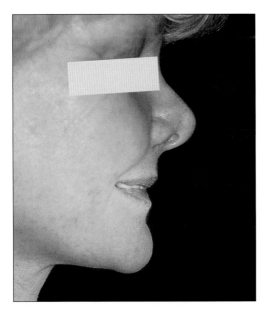

Fig 4-10 Excellent improvement in the facial esthetics, especially in the subalar base area and in the area of the reconstruction of the maxilla anteriorly. (Compare with Fig 4-1.)

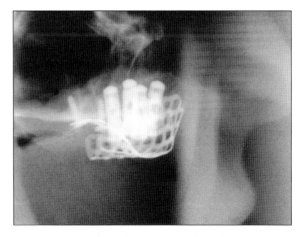

Fig 4-11 Root-form implants can be placed simultaneously with the use of the titanium mesh and the particulate autograft with Bio-Oss. Approximately 4 to 5 mm of bone exists superior to the fundi of the sockets. The implants can be stabilized, and the remainder of the root-form implant surface interfaces with the bone graft material. This procedure will be very successful, provided that the root-form implants are completely immobile.

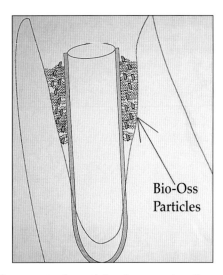 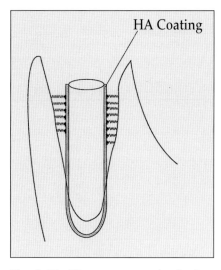

Fig 4-12 Placement of particles in an extraction socket surrounding a titanium implant. By the mechanism of conduction of bone healing between the titanium implant and the socket wall, the Bio-Oss particles (arrow) are facilitating osseous repair.

Fig 4-13 The presence of a hydroxyapatite (HA) coating on the implant surface does not appear to be a factor in facilitating bone repair or enhancing the quality of bone repair. It is the presence of particulate porous bone mineral that tends to enhance bone conduction.

One- and Two-Tooth Edentulous Defects

Techniques

The use of titanium mesh and particulate marrow and cancellous bone grafts with Bio-Oss has been very successful in smaller defects. For single-tooth replacement, the implant can be placed in the socket and the space surrounding the implant between the titanium surface and the socket wall can be grafted with porous bone mineral or other conductive materials to facilitate bone repair from the healing socket wall to the titanium surface. The placement of the conductive material also maintains the alveolar crest and facilitates the remodeling of bone in the total integration process of obtaining an optimal bone-metal interface (Figs 4-12 and 4-13).

For one- and two-tooth replacement, essentially two types of procedure can be used: immediate placement of the titanium implant at the time of the extraction of the tooth (Fig 4-14) or delayed (staged) placement of the implant after the osseous healing of the socket is completed. In the latter case, the socket is grafted with a conductive bone substitute material (eg, Bio-Oss). After approximately 3 months, the patient returns for preparation of the socket and the placement of the titanium implant (Figs 4-15 and 4-16).

In trauma cases in which the alveolar bone, especially the labial cortex, has been fractured, there may be a large deficit of the facial cortical bone. In this case, the titanium mesh is utilized to rebuild both the occlusal height of the alveolar ridge and the labial bone width (Fig 4-17).

The ideal mixture for rebuilding the labial osseous cortex in the event of fracture, avulsion, or loss of cortical bone is the patient's own par-

Fig 4-14 Immediate implant placement in a one-stage procedure immediately following tooth extraction. The area surrounding the implant is packed with porous bone mineral to facilitate the formation of bone from the socket wall to the implant surface. The titanium implant surface need not be coated with hydroxyapatite to bring about this enhancement of bone repair. The particulate conductive material (Bio-Oss) itself produces the effect. The same effect occurs in both implants coated with hydroxyapatite and those that have a titanium plasma-sprayed surface. After approximately 5 months, the implant can be uncovered and the prosthodontic restoration can be completed.

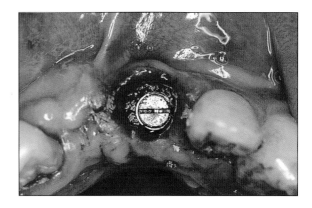

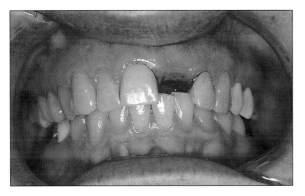

Fig 4-15 As an alternative to immediate implant placement after tooth extraction, a delayed procedure may be used. Healing is shown after the extraction of a tooth and the placement in the socket of porous bone mineral. The implant will be placed approximately 3 months after tooth extraction. The final uncovering of the implant will be 4 to 5 months later.

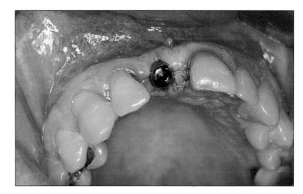

Fig 4-16 Four months following placement of the implant in a Bio-Oss–treated socket, the implant is uncovered for placement of an abutment.

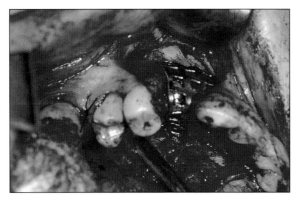

Fig 4-17 Restoration of the crestal and labial bone with TiMesh, PMCB, and Bio-Oss at the time of placement of the implant.

ticulate cancellous bone and a conductive material (ie, porous bone mineral [Bio-Oss]). The patient's own bone may be taken from the retromolar area, as previously described.

To maintain the alveolar height and prevent loss of alveolar bone height in the socket itself where the labial plate is intact, it is not necessary to use the patient's own bone as a graft in the extraction defect. The conductive porous bone mineral may be used alone in these cases and will form an excellent bony surface for the later preparation of the osteotomy to receive the titanium root-form implant; alternatively, the Bio-Oss can be placed between the titanium implant and the socket wall immediately after tooth extraction (see Fig 4-14).

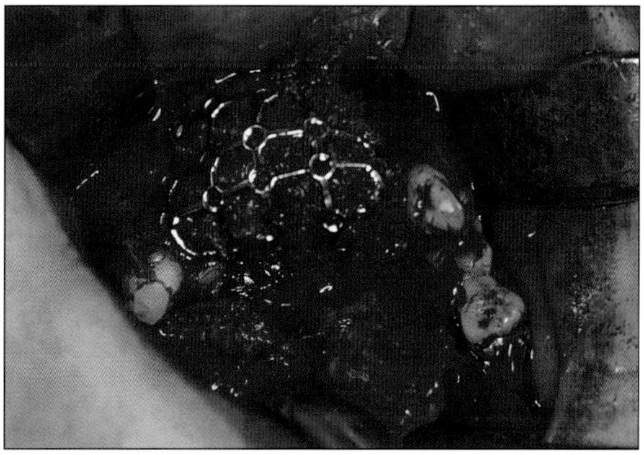

Fig 4-18 Flexible form of TiMesh. A grid form with small openings for 1.0- and 1.5-mm-diameter screws is available for use near roots of teeth. The mesh contains the graft material.

Special Materials

For the small areas presenting labial cortex fracture or avulsion, a softer titanium mesh, which is only 0.015 inch thick, may be utilized, because occlusal trauma is not a major factor in potential dislodgment or bending of the mesh while the grafted area is being remodeled over a period of approximately 4 months postoperatively.

Another type of titanium mesh, TiMesh grid (TiMesh, Inc), has both large openings and smaller grid openings for screw placement (Fig 4-18). This mesh will accommodate small, 1.0- or 1.5-mm-diameter screws. Such screws are especially useful for placement around the roots of teeth adjacent to the grafted defect or in bone adjacent to the mental foramen of the mandible (Figs 4-19a to 4-19d). Large screws are sometimes difficult to place in these areas because of their 2.2-mm diameter and the difficulty in obtaining sufficient bone to set the screw and the mesh in place without injuring adjacent tooth roots. Therefore, smaller screws (1.5 mm) and the small-grid mesh, which can be cut and adapted at the time of surgery, are usually selected for these types of defect. An appropriate microporous filter membrane may or may not be used, depending on the quality of the underlying bone, as has been discussed previously.

Fig 4-19a Use of the grid titanium mesh in the mandible near the mental foramen bilaterally. The mesh is supported by a root-form implant on one side. After remodeling of the graft, additional root-form implants are to be placed, two on each side, to support a cast bar. This type of mesh may be allowed to remain in the regenerated bone—removal is not necessary.

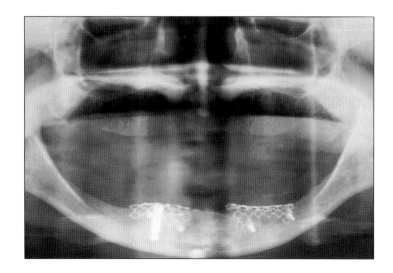

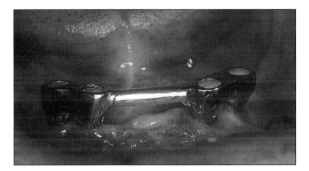

Fig 4-19b Completion of the cast bar prosthesis based on two root-form implants, which are located in the area previously grafted with PMCB and Bio-Oss. The alveolar ridge and mucosa show excellent reconstruction.

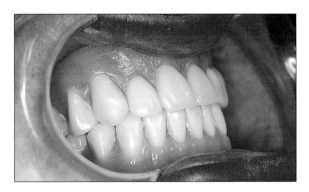

Fig 4-19c Completed mandibular and maxillary prosthesis.

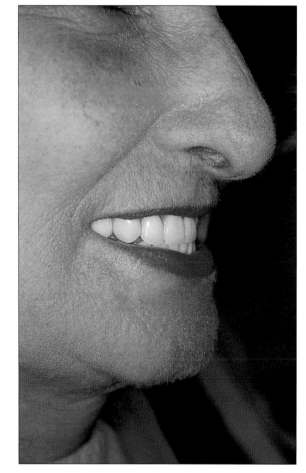

Fig 4-19d Profile of patient's prosthetic restoration.

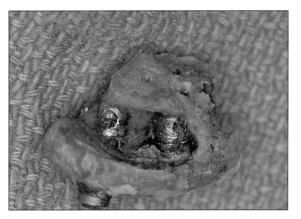 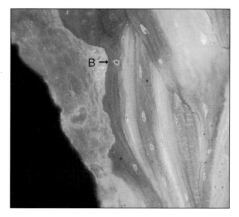

Fig 4-20 Gross specimen 6 months after placement of root-form implants in a cortical graft in a rhesus monkey so that the ends of the root-form implants were located in viable host bone. The cortical graft has undergone resorption, and large areas of the implants are in a void and not integrated. The success of such implants is due entirely to the residual host bone at the apical portion, which is holding the implants immobilized in spite of the fact that a large area of the surface of each implant is interfacing with nonviable bone.

Fig 4-21 Photomicrograph showing a root-form implant placed in the cortical bone graft in a rhesus monkey, 1 year postoperatively. A large area of nonviable cortical bone (B) is still in the area, interfering with the interfacing of the implant (shown on the left) with viable bone (original magnification ×120).

Particulate Marrow and Cancellous Bone Grafts Versus Solid Grafts

Viability

For the reconstruction of the maxilla, solid grafts may be taken autogenously from the iliac crest or from intraoral sites, such as the mentum of the mandible. However, we prefer the particulate marrow and cancellous bone grafts because this type of graft material is viable and contains a large number of pluripotential cells capable of forming bone. Cortical grafts have very few viable cells, because there are very few osteocytic and/or osteoblastic cells in the cortical portion of a cortical-cancellous block graft. When such grafts are used with implants, the graft may be pierced by the root-form titanium implants in an effort to keep them immobile. The surgeon is using a nonviable graft that, in many cases, covers approximately two thirds of the surface of the root-form implant. This nonviable graft material must undergo resorption and remodeling of bone before integration of the surface of the root-form implant can take place in that area. This repair response takes a long time postoperatively.

The particulate graft, on the other hand, can form bone de novo. While the alveolar bone is being regenerated, new bone can be integrating the root-form implant to the newly regenerated bony ridge. Thus, the process of integration of the surface of the implant is accelerated by the use of particulate grafts rather than with solid cortical-cancellous or cortical grafts. Figure 4-20 shows implants taken from a rhesus monkey 6 months after placement of the

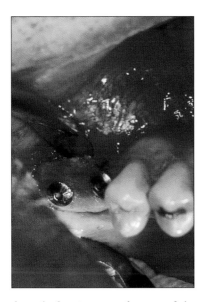

Fig 4-22a Dehisced cortical autogenous bone graft in the maxilla of a patient. The dehiscence in the mucosa has completely exposed the cortical graft. Such cortical grafts are nonviable and should be removed in the salvaging procedure. The area should be repaired with a PMCB graft.

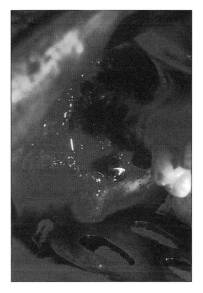

Fig 4-22b Salvaging of the implant shown in Fig 4-14a, indicating the area to be grafted with PMCB immediately next to the exposed implant. The dead cortical graft has been removed.

implants through solid bone grafts; the implants pierced the cortical autogenous free graft. The autogenous free graft is nonviable and exhibits a large area of resorption. In a photomicrograph of a similar implant from a rhesus monkey, large fragments of nonviable graft material are apparent in areas in which a significant surface of the implant is not integrated because of the presence of residual nonviable graft particles (Fig 4-21).

Response to Dehiscence

In addition, solid block nonvascularized grafts used in attempts to reconstruct the maxilla and the mandible with root-form implants do not tolerate dehiscence well. Dehiscence overlying a solid one-piece bone graft usually leads to complete loss of the graft because of the nonviability of the graft material. The graft is not able to withstand the insult of dehiscence. Figure 4-22a shows a cortical graft that had been secured with two root-form implants. Dehiscence has occurred and the entire cortical graft is exposed. The graft is a necrosed sequestrum; it must be surgically removed and the area must be regrafted if the root-form implants are to be salvaged.

If a particulate graft had been placed in such a situation, much of the particulate graft could be salvaged because of the large number of viable cells. Figure 4-22b shows the salvaging of the implants shown in Fig 4-22a. Particulate autogenous bone is used around the implant after removal of the sequestrum of the previously placed solid one-piece graft.

Integration of Root-form Implants

In experiments with rhesus monkeys, we have shown that autogenous particulate grafts placed around the surface of root-form implants readily form an interface of new bone[1] (Fig 4-23). When implants are placed through a cortical free non-revascularized bone graft, large areas of the cortical graft are still nonviable after 1 year. Figure 4-24 shows a cortical graft in a rhesus monkey. A large area of nonviable graft material is present in the area of the root-form implant. New bone is forming on the periosteal surface, but the graft material is still largely nonviable and is interfering with the integration of the root-form implant. The same phenomenon, in which there is a residual area of nonviable bone graft between the new bone and the surface of the implant, can be observed consistently in these specimens. Animal histologic evidence clearly indicates that the clinical success of grafts placed in this manner is due entirely to the residual host bone that is holding the implant in place; the rest of the surface of the implant is in jeopardy because the graft at the bone-metal interface is nonviable. Eventually, the solid nonviable graft will be remodeled and, it is hoped, replaced with new viable bone matrix, but only after a considerable time, during which the implant is at risk of being lost. The healing environment in these cases, therefore, is not as efficient as that of the PMCB-grafted root-form implant.

Our system is versatile and adaptable to many types of cases. The titanium mesh with the root-form implants can be placed at the time of the placement of the graft or in a delayed or staged procedure in which the root-form implants are placed later. The use of bone-conductive Bio-Oss porous bone mineral with PMCB to restore edentulous areas of the mandible and maxilla for both conventional and implant-borne prostheses is shown in Figs 4-25a to 4-25h.

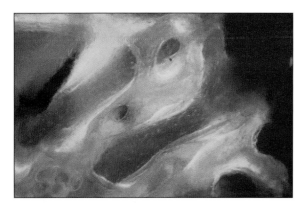

Fig 4-23 Titanium implant–graft interface in a rhesus monkey in which a PMCB graft was used. Viable bone (left) is seen along the entire length of the interface between the implant (far right) and the PMCB graft. This is in contrast to an implant placed in a cortical bone graft, in which there is no viable new bone next to the implant surface until the cortical graft has been completely resorbed and remodeled (original magnification ×40).

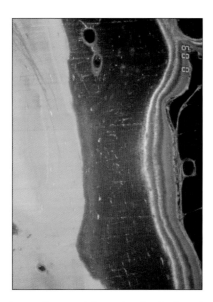

Fig 4-24 Interface of a root-form implant placed through a large residual segment of nonviable cortical bone (light area) from an autogenous graft used in a rhesus monkey. One year after grafting, a large area of nonviable bone is still present next to the root-form implant, which is at the far left margin. Two increments of new periosteal bone have been labeled by intravitally administered tetracycline (far right), but the large sequestrum from the original graft is preventing new bone from reaching the implant.

Fig 4-25a Bone loss radiographic characteristics of the combination syndrome, in which there is marked atrophy of bone in the posterior area of the mandible because of the prolonged retention of the anterior teeth and use of a free-end saddle prosthesis. There is also marked loss of bone in the anterior part of the maxilla because the natural teeth of the mandible have been occluding against an unstable maxillary denture.

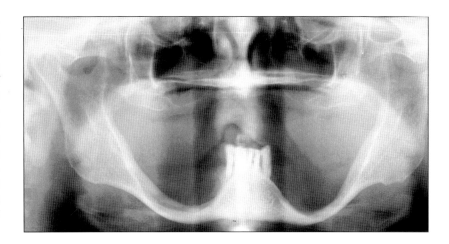

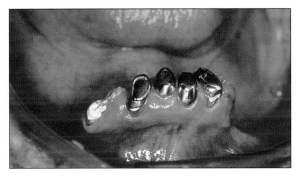

Fig 4-25b Clinical view of a similar case of combination syndrome shows the level of bone around the anterior teeth of the mandible, which have been in function for a long time while the posterior teeth have been missing and restored with a free-end saddle prosthesis.

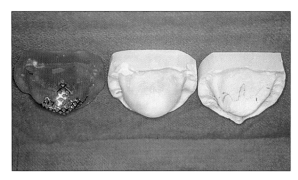

Fig 4-25c Cast of a maxilla with the anterior waxup and the secondary acrylic resin cast for the formation of a titanium mesh carrier for PMCB and Bio-Oss reconstruction of the maxilla (for the case shown in Figs 4-25d to 4-25h).

Fig 4-25d Titanium mesh in place in the maxilla. The natural teeth in the anterior mandibular are retained. Appropriate occlusion must be well stabilized and maintained postoperatively with the new prosthesis to prevent a repetition of the bone loss in the anterior part of the maxilla.

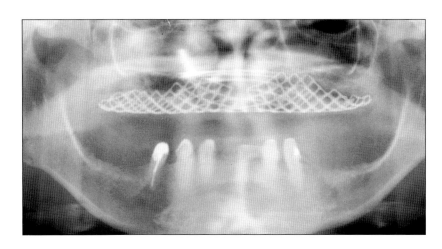

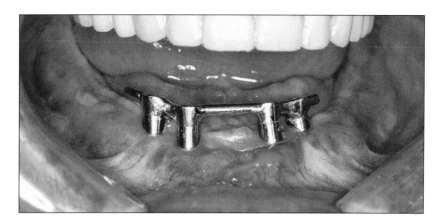

Fig 4-25e Bar implant-supported prosthesis on the mandible against a maxillary conventional complete denture. This type of prosthesis may produce the same type of atrophy in the anterior part of the maxilla as is produced by prolonged retention of the natural mandibular anterior teeth, if the occlusion of the prosthesis is not well monitored.

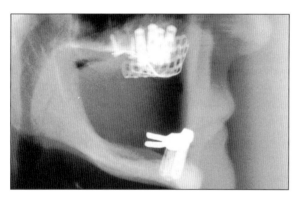

Fig 4-25f Anterior maxillary bone loss has occurred 1 1/2 years after mandibular implant placement. Treatment of such bone loss of the anterior maxilla is shown. Titanium mesh with a PMCB graft has been placed in the anterior part of the maxilla, and root-form implants have been placed concomitantly. At the same time, the mandibular implant-supported prosthesis has been retained to produce the final effect of implant-supported prostheses in both the maxillary and mandibular arches.

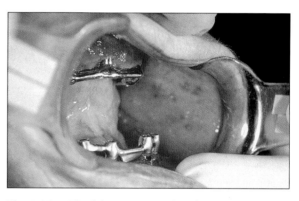

Fig 4-25g Final bar construction for implant-borne prostheses in both the maxilla and the mandible.

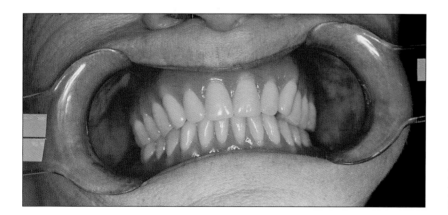

Fig 4-25h Final implant-borne prostheses for both maxilla and mandible.

Clinical cases correlate well with data from rhesus monkeys, which demonstrate excellent bone remodeling around root-form implants in full function (Figs 4-26a and 4-26b).

We have been using this system of titanium mesh with the Bio-Oss combination for root-form implants over a 6-year period. Among a total of 50 patients and 290 implants in the maxilla, we have observed no patient failures involving four implants during this time. Restoration of both bone height and bone width has been excellent in all patients, and the character of the bone surrounding the implants is exceptional; bone density is good throughout the grafted implant and bony areas.

Advantages of the Titanium Mesh–Composite Graft Technique

Use of the TiMesh with PMCB and Bio-Oss grafting instead of block one-piece grafting has several advantages:

1. The titanium mesh system is simple and straightforward and can be adjusted to individual requirements.
2. Physiologic bone remodeling occurs following the grafting procedure. Such remodeling and replacement of the graft with viable bone is very slow when a block one-piece cortical autogenous graft is used, but very rapid and complete with a PMCB graft.

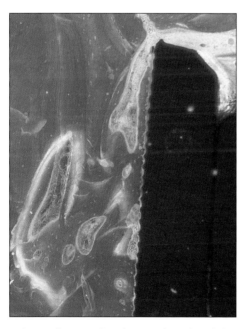

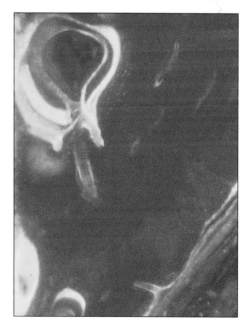

Fig 4-26a Photomicrograph taken under ultraviolet light showing new bone formation labeled by tetracycline around an implant on a fixed prosthesis in a rhesus monkey. The implant had been full function for 1.5 years. Changes in the surrounding trabecular pattern are shown. The Bio-Oss particles placed at the same time as the root-form implant have been, for the most part, remodeled to form a dense trabecular pattern and lamellar bone.

Fig 4-26b Same type of response from a rhesus monkey mandible having root-form implants and Bio-Oss in full function for 1 1/2 years. This is the healthy response of the trabecular bone to changes in function. Where there is very thin trabecular bone, a sudden change in occlusal force may result in the lessening of the bone formation along the implant surface. Thickening of the trabecular pattern and cortex remodeling are indications of appropriate bone response (original magnification ×100).

3. The area, size, and contour of the bone regeneration is dictated by the size and shape of the titanium mesh, and the height and width of the regenerated alveolar bone can be controlled very precisely. In contrast, the area, contour, and size of the solid grafted areas are very difficult to control because of the inherent shape of the cortical or cortical-cancellous bone graft itself, which must be fashioned to fit the contours and curves of the mandible and maxilla.
4. The technique is very predictable, as shown by long-term analysis of our cases.
5. There is no need for subsequent or multiple procedures for vestibuloplasty, because the vestibular height is established at the time of removal of the titanium mesh.
6. There is no need for use of remote flaps or extensive soft-tissue surgery.

Reference

1. Boyne PJ. Analysis of performance of root-form endosseous implants placed in the maxillary sinus. J Long-Term Effects Med Implants 1993;3:143–159.

Chapter 5

After Combination Syndrome, Trauma, or Oncologic Surgery

Treatment of Combination Syndrome

The term *combination syndrome* is used to describe the loss of anterior maxillary bone and posterior mandibular bone that results from prolonged use of a mandibular free-end saddle prosthesis with retention of the natural mandibular anterior teeth against a maxillary conventional complete denture. The mandibular anterior natural teeth place inappropriate functional forces on the anterior part of the maxilla, resulting in loss of bone in the region. This is particularly true when an unstable occlusion is superimposed on the anatomically unfavorable alveolar ridge. The inherent instability of the free-end saddle prosthesis also tends to cause loss of bone in the posterior portion of the mandible (see Figs 4-25a to 4-25d).

We address this problem by utilizing a posterior particulate marrow and cancellous bone (PMCB) graft, with or without posterior root-form implants, in the mandible and by using PMCB graft in a titanium mesh carrier to restore the maxillary anterior ridge. We have found that this technique can produce good results with root-form implants placed in the anterior maxilla in a staged or immediate procedure.

However, a variation of the combination syndrome can be produced iatrogenically when an atrophic mandible is restored with a bar implant-supported prosthesis occluding against a maxillary conventional complete denture (see Fig 4-25e). The increased function afforded by the implant-borne mandibular denture against the maxillary conventional complete denture over a period of 2 to 4 years can lead to resorption of the anterior maxilla, especially in those cases in which there is difficulty in obtaining good occlusal contact, good occlusal function, and proper incisal relationship.

This condition can result in the need to augment the anterior maxilla with a bone graft and remake the maxillary prosthesis. Accordingly, we utilize titanium mesh with the immediate placement, wherever possible, of root-form implants in a one-staged procedure (see Fig 4-25f). After 5 months, the mesh is removed and the implants are uncovered for placement of the healing abutments and fabrication of the complete denture (see Figs 4-25g and 4-25h).

Because this maxillary anterior bone loss has a tendency to develop, if a Dolder bar prosthesis is used in the mandible in patients having a long-standing completely edentulous maxilla, we place a root-form implant–supported maxillary prosthesis as well. This equalizes the forces to be applied to the anterior maxilla, stabilizing occlusal function so that an implant-borne prosthesis exists on both maxilla and mandible. When this is done, there is no resorption of the anterior maxillary ridge (see Figs 4-25e to 4-25h). In these cases, Bio-Oss particulate bone mineral (Geistlich Sons/Osteohealth Co) is also used to increase the bone density, which also aids in aborting further resorption of the anterior maxilla.

Increasing Bone Density

The previously described technique has the built-in advantage of increasing the bone density in areas of restored bone and around root-form implants. The concept of increasing bone density has been the result of work with rhesus monkeys, in which root-form implants have been placed in extraction sockets at the time the teeth are extracted (see Figs 4-26a and 4-26b). Bio-Oss has been placed surrounding implants between the implant surface and the wall of the socket.

In clinical practice, root-form implants may be placed in fresh extraction sockets or placed as a delayed procedure in healed sockets that were grafted with Bio-Oss at the time of extraction (see Figs 4-12 to 4-16). Titanium mesh may also be used to reconstruct the labial plate after tooth extraction (see Figs 4-17 to 4-19). Porous bone mineral placed at the interface between the titanium implants and bony socket wall has been shown to:

1. Enhance the rate of bone formation between the socket wall and the titanium implant surface to maintain the alveolar ridge height at the crest of the ridge surrounding the extraction socket.
2. Create an environment for a maximally effective bone response to functional changes occurring in occlusal loading.
3. Produce changes in the trabecular pattern of both the posterior and the anterior parts of the maxilla. The fine trabecular pattern with large areas of vascular marrow spaces found in these areas of the maxilla is changed to one of increased bone density and a thickened trabecular pattern. This change tends to enhance the amount of osseous matrix at the bone interface of root-form implants over a long period of time and to decrease the possibility of alveolar ridge bone resorption.

Root-form implants have been placed as a staged procedure after implantation of the extraction sockets of Macaca fascicularis with Bio-Oss (Figs 5-1a to 5-1c). The ridges were allowed to mature for 2 months before titanium implants were placed. Titanium implants were used for complete-denture prostheses. An alveolar bone maintenance phenomenon has been demonstrated by placing rhesus monkeys in occlusal function with implant-supported prostheses (Figs 5-1d to 5-1f). The result was excellent maintenance of the alveolar bone without loosening or loss of implants, without formation of periodontal pockets, and with excellent function over an 18-month period. (In human chronology, this period is equal to 3 to 4 years of clinical function.) Such work demonstrates the concept that an increase in bone density is favorable to long-term occlusal and prosthetic function.

An example of the bone interface response around root-form implants placed in Bio-Oss–implanted sockets is shown in Fig 5-1g. There are areas of increased bone density at the titanium surface, showing response to the

Fig 5-1a to 5-1g Macaca fascicularis with an implant-supported prosthesis in function for 18 months. The prosthesis was based on Bio-Oss–implanted sockets in which implants were placed 2 months postextraction. A complete denture was constructed and in place for 18 months with excellent clinical and radiographic results.

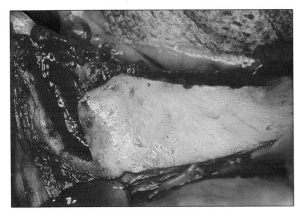

Fig 5-1a Surgical defect after extraction of the posterior teeth in a mature Macaca fascicularis.

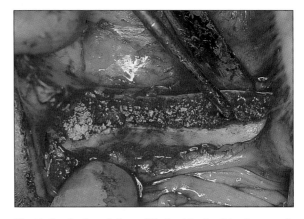

Fig 5-1b Socket defects filled with the Bio-Oss particles.

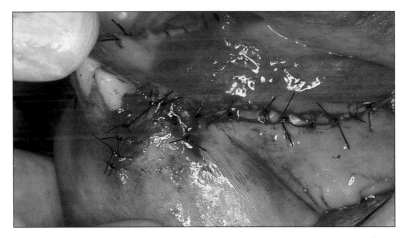

Fig 5-1c Closure of the mucoperiosteum.

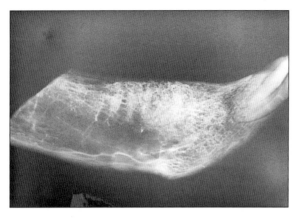

Fig 5-1d Increased bone density 6 months after tooth extraction and placement of Bio-Oss.

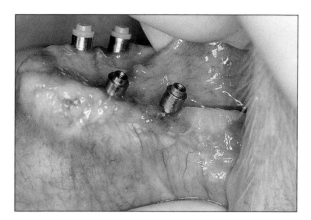

Fig 5-1e Root-form implants, which are here uncovered for placement of abutments.

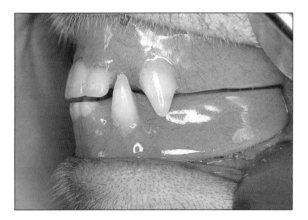

Fig 5-1f Complete dentures in place. The dentures were in function for 18 months.

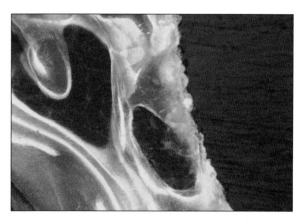

Fig 5-1g Ground section of one of the implants that was in function for 18 months. Ultraviolet microscopy shows concentration of bone around the implant apex (original magnification ×150).

stimuli of 18 months of full function in adult Macaca fascicularis.

In addition, we have long-term studies of conventional prostheses[1] placed over atrophic mandibles in clinical patients whose alveolar ridges have been restored with particulate marrow and cancellous bone and porous bone mineral (Bio-Oss)[1] (Figs 5-2a to 5-2d). Conventional prostheses placed over such grafted areas and in full function for a period of 5 years have exhibited only a 25% loss of alveolar bone height,[1] indicating that the increased bone density, even under conventional prostheses, is producing an environment that is resistant to the resorptive processes that normally occur. This study has now been extended to an 8- to 9-year period, and excellent results have been reported; less than 30% of bone height of the alveolar ridge has been lost over the 9-year follow-up period.

Fig 5-2a Mandibular atrophy, resulting in marked bone loss. The atrophy will be treated with bone grafts of Bio-Oss and PMCB.

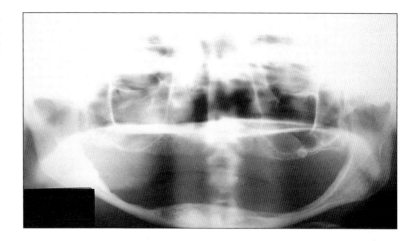

Fig 5-2b Mandibular atrophy treated by PMCB and Bio-Oss. Bone maintenance after 5 years is excellent.

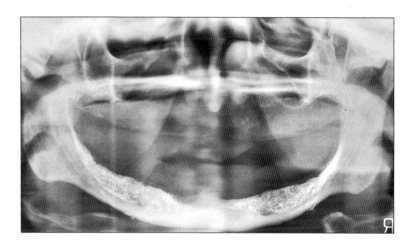

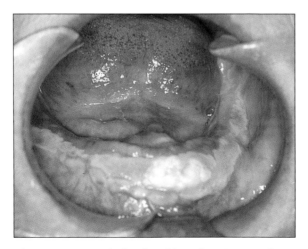

Fig 5-2c Restored alveolar ridge after 5 years, showing excellent maintenance.

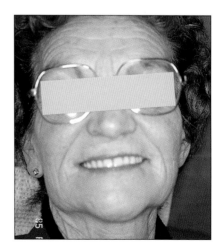

Fig 5-2d Patient with conventional complete prosthesis after 5 years of functioning on the restored ridges.

Special Considerations for the Mandible

While the titanium mesh of 0.020-inch thickness may be used effectively in the total and subtotal maxilla, its use for reconstruction of the entire mandible is not as productive. When placed over an entire atrophic mandible, the large area of titanium mesh may lead to dehiscence due to the thinness of the mucosa over the posterior mandibular ridge and other anatomic features of the mandible itself.

Partially edentulous areas of the mandible, however, may be treated with the 0.020-inch thick mesh very effectively (Figs 5-3a and 5-3b). A more effective method of treating partially edentulous areas involves the use of the grid mesh (TiMesh grid; TiMesh, Inc), which is thinner and flexible, and can be adapted at surgery using the small titanium screws to effectively secure the mesh avoiding the roots of the adjacent teeth. The outline and contour of the desired height and width of the reconstruction will be determined by the contour and size of the grid mesh. The usual mixture of Bio-Oss and the patient's own bone, PMCB, is used in these areas. The effective use of the grid mesh in the mandible especially in the anterior as well on the posterior aspect roughly parallels that of its use in the maxilla (Figs 5-4a and 5-4b; see Figs 4-19a to 4-19c).

Rather than using the 0.020-inch thick titanium mesh in treating atrophy of the posterior mandible, we use a technique involving an iliac crest cortical graft approximately 2.5 x 5 cm on the lingual surface only of the thin mandible.[1,2] This cortical "strut" graft is secured with circummandibular wires. The cortical graft or strut serves as a wall against which the graft of the 50/50 mix of Bio-Oss and PMCB is placed (Figs 5-5a to 5-5g). This procedure has been shown to be very effective for conventional dentures.[1,2]

Now the same technique is used with a staged placement of root-form implants with high degree of success. Figures 5-6a to 5-6e show a case after 10 years of function using a mandibular tissue bar placed on four IMZ implants in a graft composed of 50/50 mixture of autogenous cancellous bone PMCB from the iliac crest, and porous bone mineral product similar to Bio-Oss. Thus the described concept of grafting can be applied to the mandible with modifications for the anatomic features involved.

Special Considerations for the Mandible

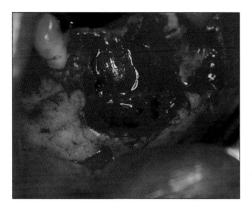

Fig 5-3a Intraoperative view of a mandibular anterior defect in the symphyseal area following the resection of a benign tumor. Both lingual and buccal cortices have been resected and the defect requires the reconstruction of ridge thickness and height of the ridge at the labial and lingual crest.

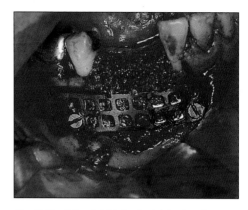

Fig 5-3b The 0.020-inch thick titanium mesh is used in this case since the area is sufficiently large to accept the large diameter size of screws. The titanium mesh is positioned to avoid encroachment upon the mental foramen. The mental nerve is on the lower left portion of the slide.

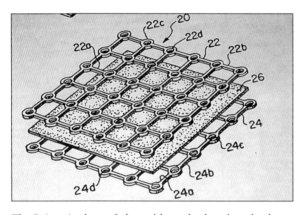

Fig 5-4a A view of the grid mesh showing the large mesh openings and the small openings to accommodate the 1 mm size titanium screws.

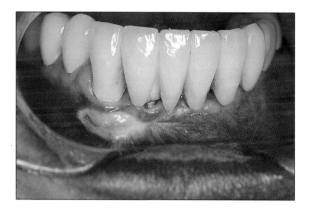

Fig 5-4b A case in which the grid mesh has been used to restore an anterior mandibular deficient area prior to placing implants for the prosthesis. There is excellent width and good vestibular height. A palatal patch graft has been placed at the lower left cuspid vestibule (white area) to relieve a high soft tissue attachment. The appropriate height and width has been restored by this procedure and the use of the fine grid mesh. This type of grid mesh was also used in the case shown in Figs 4-19a to 4-19c.

After Combination Syndrome, Trauma, or Oncologic Surgery

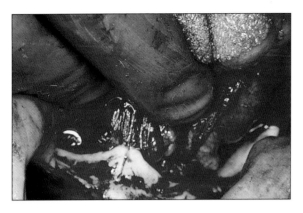

Fig 5-5a An intraoperative view of a markedly atrophic mandible following the elevation of the mucoperiosteal flaps. The genial tubercle is prominent anteriorly and the area of excessive atrophy is located in the posterior aspect of the mandible bilaterally.

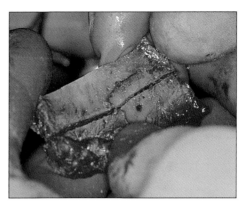

Fig 5-5b Shows a cortical cancellous graft taken from the lateral table of the anterior iliac crest. This will be cut into two "struts," 5.5 cm long × 2 cm high. The initial cut to produce one of these "struts" is shown here. Holes are then placed in the strut, which is placed on lingual surface of the mandible posteriorly.

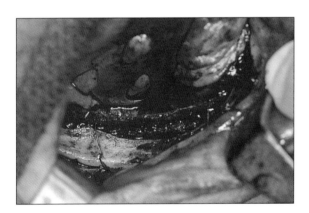

Fig 5-5c Shows a cortical "strut" placed along the lingual aspect of the atrophic mandibular ridge. An additional strut will be placed on the contralateral lingual side, and maintained by circummandibular wires.

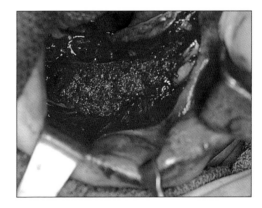

Fig 5-5d Shows the placement of the autogenous bone and the Bio-Oss against the lingually placed cortical autogenous strut. This placement of bone in this manner serves to move the crest of the atrophic, mandibular ridge lingually where it formally existed prior to the severe bone loss from atrophy.

Special Considerations for the Mandible

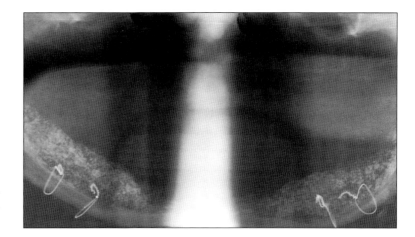

Fig 5-5e Shows the immediate postoperative radiographs with the circummandibular wires in place.

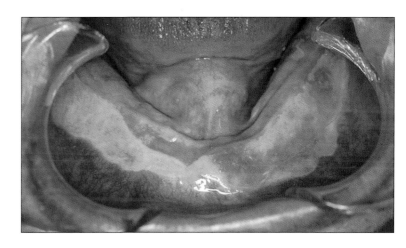

Fig 5-5f The clinical view 4 months postoperatively after a split-thickness skin graft to restore the buccal vestibule for conventional prosthesis. Note that the crest of the ridge has been returned to a more lingual position in concert with the maxillary edentulous alveolar crest.

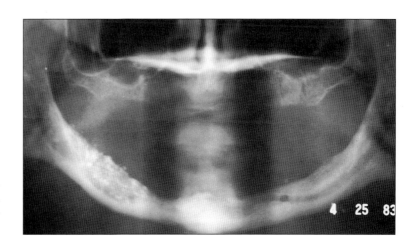

Fig 5-5g Radiographs 5 years postoperatively showing excellent maintenance of the alveolar ridge under conventional prosthodontic function.

After Combination Syndrome, Trauma, or Oncologic Surgery

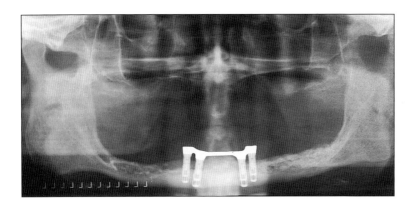

Fig 5-6a Radiographic view of four IMZ implants placed 10 years previously in an extremely atrophic mandible which was grafted with an anorganic porous bone mineral product, very similar to Bio-Oss. The augmented height of the ridge can be seen maintaining its height and width over the 10-year period.

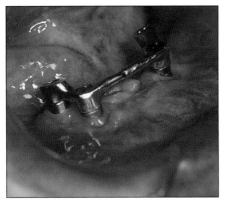

Fig 5-6b Clinical view of the excellent tissue response around the individually placed implants at the 10-year follow-up examination. The maximum probed pocket depth was 2 to 2.5 mm and the tissue was in excellent health.

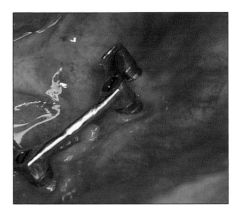

Fig 5-6c Another view of the implant bar showing excellent tissue tone.

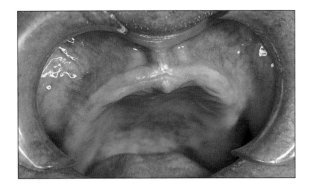

Fig 5-6d Shows the maxillary ridge indicating that there has been no loss of the maxillary bone. The excellent occlusion has prevented maxillary bone loss.

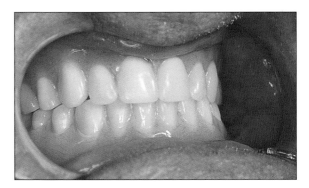

Fig 5-6e The occlusion 10 years after surgery with good balance and no excessive force in the incisor contact area. This case indicates the ability of porous bone mineral to maintain restored grafted areas in the mandible under appropriate prosthodontic function.

Use as a Barrier

It is not widely understood that materials other than membranes can serve as barriers to the ingrowth of fibrous connective tissue into bony areas that have been grafted or that are undergoing healing and regeneration. Conductive bone graft substitute materials, if properly accepted in the organized clot and properly utilized in the bone-grafted area, will contribute to the remodeling process and will inhibit the ingress and ingrowth of fibrous connective tissue and the downgrowth of epithelium from the surface of the mucosa. It has been shown histologically from our animal specimens that this "barrier" phenomenon occurs.

Clinical evidence also demonstrates the barrier effect of a mixture of porous bone mineral and the patient's own bone (as a graft) in stopping connective tissue from inhibiting bone regeneration (Figs 5-7a to 5-7d). Figures 5-7a to 5-7d illustrate regeneration of a large periodontal area of the buccal cortex, the lateral cortical bone defect, and the periapical defect.

Figs 5-7a to 5-7d Barrier capabilities of the mixture of PMCB and conductive material (Bio-Oss).

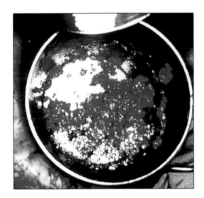

Fig 5-7a Mixture of particulate marrow and cancellous bone and Bio-Oss. This type of graft material is capable of producing an occlusive barrier to the host connective tissue, allowing bone to repair with an excellent cortical surface.

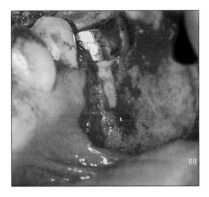

Fig 5-7b Molar tooth with a fractured root, periodontal bone loss, periapical bone loss, and marked loss of bone along the buccal aspect of the cortical portion of the alveolar ridge. This was treated with extraction of the tooth and the immediate placement of the implant.

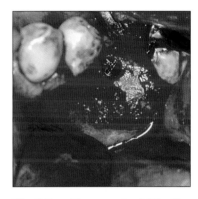

Fig 5-7c Placement of Bio-Oss and PMCB in the cortical periapical, periodontal, and crestal defects.

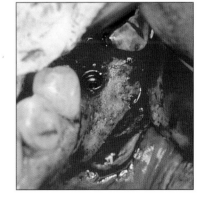

Fig 5-7d Same patient 5 months after grafting. The elevation of the mucoperiosteal flap reveals re-formation of the cortical plate, complete regeneration of the periapical and periodontal bone, good formation of new bone, and maintenance of new bone at the labial crest. The maintenance of bone at the labial crest and the regeneration of bone in this manner do not necessarily require a membrane system for guided tissue regeneration. A conductive material (Bio-Oss), used appropriately, can also serve as a barrier.

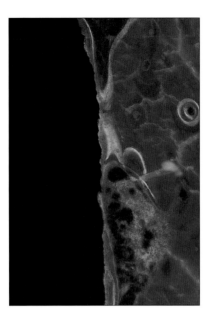

Fig 5-8 Histologic specimen from a Rhesus monkey showing a defect similar to that shown in Fig 5-7 in which a mixture of autogenous particles and Bio-Oss had been placed in a lateral alveolar mandibular defect to support a root-form implant. The outer periosteal surface (left center) shows good cortical bone having formed along the ridge 4 months postgrafting illustrating the "barrier effect" of such a composite graft.

Figure 5-7d shows the crestal bone and buccal bone 5 months after the use of a mixture of the patient's own bone and porous bone mineral in approximately a 50-50 mixture. Thus we have both clinical and animal experimental histologic evidence that conductive material can serve effectively as a barrier (Fig 5-8).

In general, materials that serve best in this manner are those that are slowly resorbed (eg, Bio-Oss). Materials that are completely unresorbable, such as HTR (Bioplant), may have a similar effect, although the bone response is not as complete in its barrier potential as is a conductive graft material such as Bio-Oss, which slowly undergoes remodeling and incorporation into the graft and assists in the formation of a new bony cortex.

Reconstruction Following Trauma and Oncologic Surgery

Hemimaxillectomies and other partial maxillary resections for oncologic surgery procedures leave large deficits of the maxilla. In the past, these have been very difficult to address because of the anatomy of the maxilla and the difficulty in obtaining properly sized grafts and proper contours for the area to be grafted. We have been able to apply this technique to extend titanium mesh over the buttress of the zygoma and across the palate to the contralateral side in patients who have undergone hemimaxillectomies or experienced partial traumatic avulsion of the maxilla. This technique has produced excellent osseous reconstruction of both the maxilla and mandible and has enhanced the ability of the surgeon to produce not only osseous reconstruction but also quality prosthetic reconstruction, in the form of root-form implant–borne prostheses.

Cases are presented to demonstrate the use of this technique in large defects involving traumatic loss of the mandible and maxilla as well as postoncologic surgery defects.

Figures 5-9 and 5-10 show reconstruction of the mandible after massive tissue loss from gunshot wounds. Figures 5-11a to 5-11e show the same techniques applied to reconstruction of a postoncologic surgical defect.

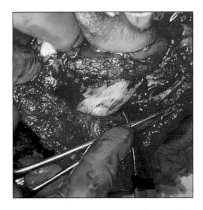

Fig 5-9a Reconstruction of a mandible following a gunshot wound that resulted in loss of the mandibular body on the right side. Intraoperative view of the avulsive wound, revealing severe comminution of the mandible.

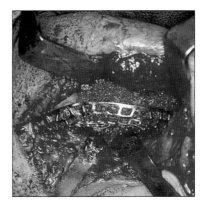

Fig 5-9b Placement of the iliac crest PMCB and Bio-Oss graft in a titanium mesh.

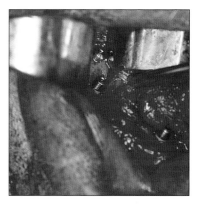

Fig 5-9c Placement of the root-form implants after maturation and remodeling of the graft.

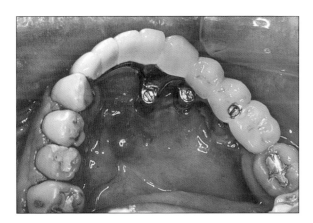

Fig 5-9d Completed prosthesis.

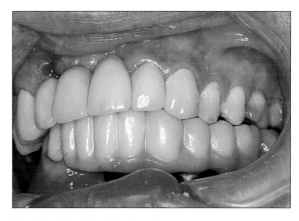

Fig 5-9e Prosthesis in function.

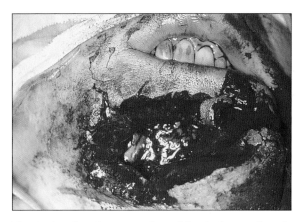

Fig 5-10a Gunshot wound resulting in loss and avulsion of the anterior and right body of the mandible.

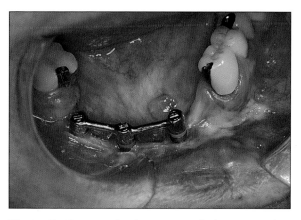

Fig 5-10b Bar prosthesis, connected after restoration of the defect with PMCB and Bio-Oss and placement of implants in a titanium orthopedic mesh.

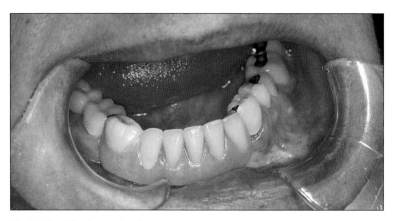

Fig 5-10c Final prosthesis.

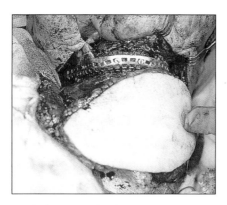

Fig 5-11a Loss of the entire body of the mandible due to osteoradionecrosis following irradiation for carcinoma of the floor of the mouth and mandible. TiMesh full mandible has been packed with PMCB and Bio-Oss. A free flap is visible below the titanium mesh.

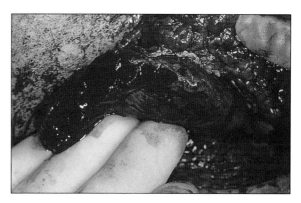

Fig 5-11b A free soft-tissue flap is brought up from the musculus rectus abdominis and is made to cover the graft with microvascular anastomosis to the superior thyroid vessels. This type of soft-tissue graft enhances the vascular perfusion of the PMCB graft in compromised cases, eg, postirradiation deficits.

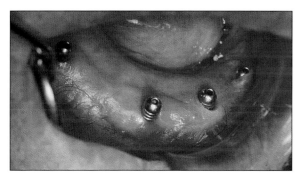

Fig 5-11c After integration of the implants, which were placed 5 months after bone grafting, selected implants have been uncovered and abutments have been placed.

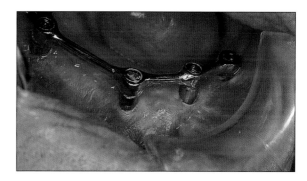

Fig 5-11d Implant bar prosthesis.

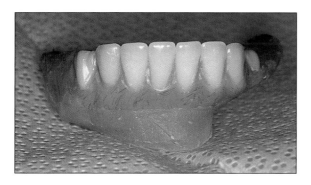

Fig 5-11e Final prosthesis.

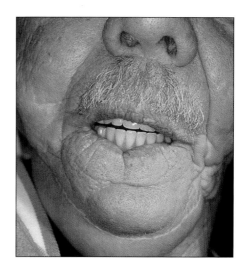

Figs 5-12a to 5-12e Reconstruction of an entire maxilla presenting with massive bone loss from atrophy and infection following use of three subperiosteal implants.

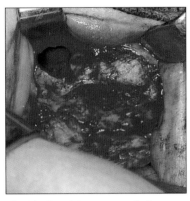

Fig 5-12a Exposure of the premaxilla reveals complete atrophy. Some hydroxyapatite is visible in the floor of the nose, and the lateral antral wall is exposed by bone atrophy. The defects are similar to those of traumatic origin.

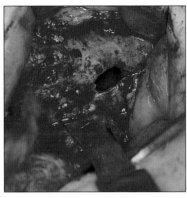

Fig 5-12b Large opening into the floor of the nose and another palatal opening into the left antrum.

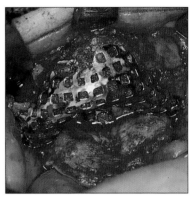

Fig 5-12c TiMesh, with graft of PMCB and Bio-Oss, in place.

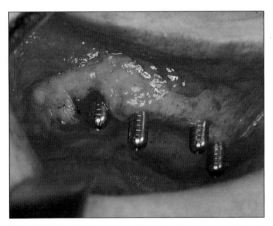

Fig 5-12d Abutments placed after 5 months of integration of the implants, which were inserted when the titanium mesh was removed, 5 months after grafting.

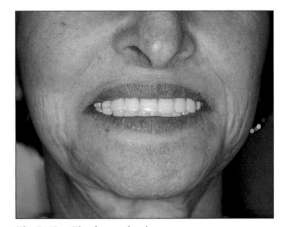

Fig 5-12e Final prosthesis.

Figures 5-12 and 5-13 illustrate the use of titanium mesh in reconstruction of maxillas lost as a result of atrophy and infection. In this latter category, we have followed for a period of over 5 years a series of 39 patients whose maxillas have been restored with the same technique. In the patient shown in Figs 5-12a to 5-12e, both antra and the nasal floor are exposed by atrophy of the bone. In the patient shown in Figs 5-13a to 5-13h, previous use of hydroxyapatite in a particulate solid form in an attempt to restore the lost ridge has led to extensive bone loss. The hydroxyapatite in such cases must be completely removed to obtain healthy bone for placement of root-form implants. Figures 5-14a to 5-14i show the placement of root-form implants in a deficient atrophic premaxilla secondary to comminuted fracture sustained by the patient.

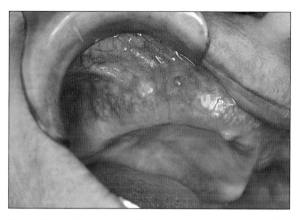

Fig 5-13a Massive maxillary atrophy occurring after hydroxyapatite had been placed 2 years previously. The hydroxyapatite particles were mobile, causing the patient pain on use of a conventional denture. The bulging ridge is shown with the mucosa stretched over the hydroxyapatite.

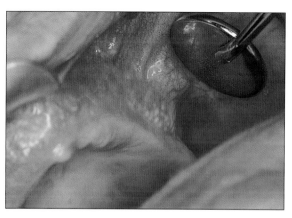

Fig 5-13b Mass of hydroxyapatite beneath the mucosa displaced laterally onto the zygomatic buttress.

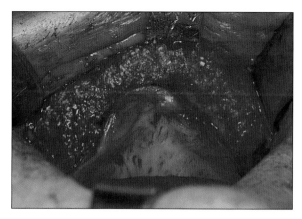

Fig 5-13c View after exposure of the maxilla prior to removal of the hydroxyapatite particles.

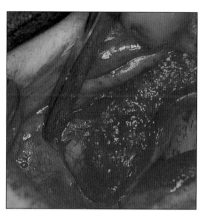

Fig 5-13d View of the hydroxyapatite particles displaced laterally to the right zygomatic buttress.

After Combination Syndrome, Trauma, or Oncologic Surgery

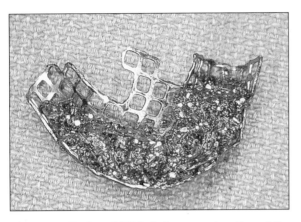

Fig 5-13e Graft and TiMesh for reconstruction of the maxilla after removal of the hydroxyapatite. The surgical site resembled a post-traumatic defect.

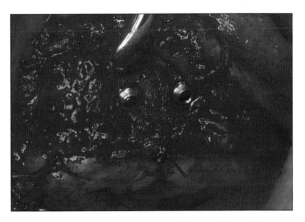

Fig 5-13f Reconstructed maxillary ridge after removal of the titanium mesh 5 months after grafting. Thickness, width, and height of the ridge are excellent. Root-form implants are being placed at the same time that the TiMesh is being removed.

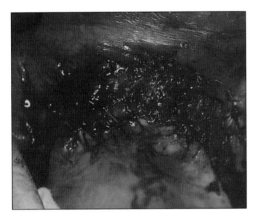

Fig 5-13g Reconstruction of the vestibule after removal of the TiMesh and placement of the root-form implants.

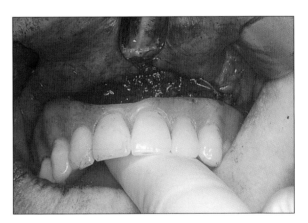

Figs 5-13h Adjustment of the previous prosthesis to support the new vestibule as a splint. The increase in vestibular height is appreciable.

Figs 5-14a to 5-14i Another case demonstrating a fracture comminution of the maxilla sustained in a motor vehicle accident. The alveolar ridge was extremely thin and almost nonexistent on the left side.

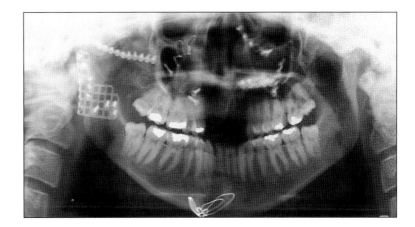

Fig 5-14a Radiograph showing multiple facial injuries, including avulsion and comminution of the anterior maxilla.

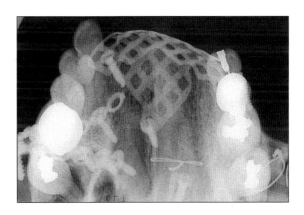

Fig 5-14b Radiograph showing the titanium mesh with the PMCB and Bio-Oss graft to reconstruct the premaxilla.

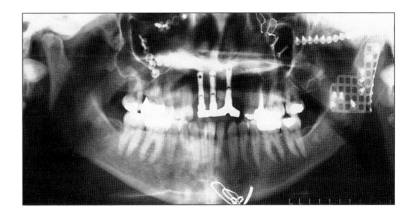

Fig 5-14c Radiograph showing the implants in place after removal of the TiMesh. The middle implant is in the midline of the maxilla because there is more residual bone in that area. The implant on the left is also in the maximum area of bone available.

After Combination Syndrome, Trauma, or Oncologic Surgery

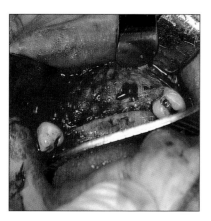

Fig 5-14d View after the removal of the titanium mesh and creation of the new vestibule revealing the new vestibular height.

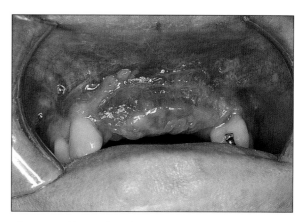

Fig 5-14e Six weeks after removal of the TiMesh. The attached mucosa has re-formed by reepithelializing the denuded area remaining after the vestibuloplasty.

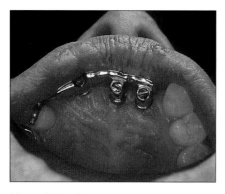

Fig 5-14f Position of the abutments. The implant and abutment to replace the central incisors are positioned in the maxillary midline to take advantage of the maximum bone support.

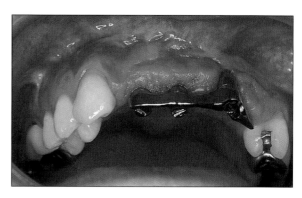

Fig 5-14g Bar prosthesis in place. The implants have excellent osseous support.

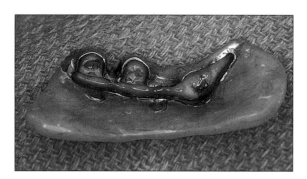

Fig 5-14h Completed prosthesis.

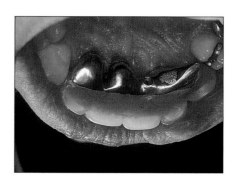

Fig 5-14i Prosthesis in place.

Titanium mesh may also be used with free flaps (microvascular anastomosis) (Figs 5-15 and 5-16). In free fibular grafts with microvascular anastomosis, implants may be placed simultaneously with the bone graft or approximately 6 months later, usually in conjunction with an augmentation PMCB graft to afford additional bony support for the root-form implants.

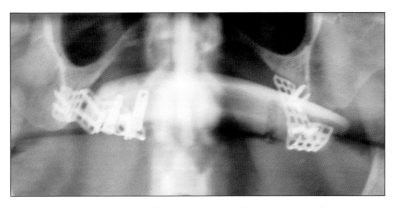

Fig 5-15 Reconstruction of a resected maxilla with a free flap from the fibula. Titanium mesh is attaching the free graft to the zygomatic buttresses bilaterally. Two root-form implants were placed on one side at the time of graft placement; two additional implants will be placed later to avoid pressure at the time of surgery on the pedicle and blood supply.

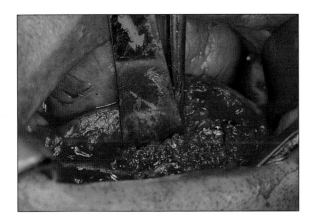
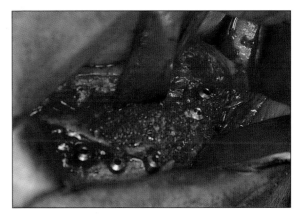

Fig 5-16 Fibular free-flap graft restoring a mandible that had been avulsed by gunshot wound. Particulate marrow and cancellous bone from the iliac crest is placed over the fibula to provide additional bone support for the root-form implants, which are being placed approximately 5 months after the original free flap surgery.

References

1. Boyne PJ. Vergleich von Bio-Oss und anderen Implantationsmaterialien bei der Erhaltung des Alveolarkammes des Unterkiefers beim Menschen. Unfallheilkunde 1991;216:98–103.
2. Boyne PJ, James RA. Research in subperiosteal implant surgery. In: Hardin JF (ed). Clark's Clinical Dentistry. Philadelphia: Lippincott, 1987.

Chapter 6

For Treatment of Maxillary Clefts

Three important principles of successful bone grafting in cleft palates involve the proper selection of the appropriate bone grafting material; the sequencing of alveolar cleft grafting with orthodontic treatment, appropriate application of orthopedic forces to produce and maintain normal growth of the maxilla; and the use of maximally effective root-form implants and a prosthesis to ensure maintenance of the grafted area and full function.

Historically, bone grafting for treatment of cleft palate involved the use of ribs and other cortical grafts or solid one-piece cortical cancellous grafts. Such grafts were used between 1950 and 1970, particularly in Europe.

However, poor results from these surgical procedures led to an almost complete cessation of the use of grafting to treat clefts, primarily because of the effect the cortical-cancellous rib graft on the growth of the child. This type of grafting tended to result in resorption of the graft and residual scar formation in the operated cleft areas. The graft resorption left fibrous tissue that tended to interfere with the growth patterns of the maxilla.

Figure 6-1, showing the failure of a cortical one-piece graft in a premaxillary cleft, reveals an almost complete loss of the graft, inappro-

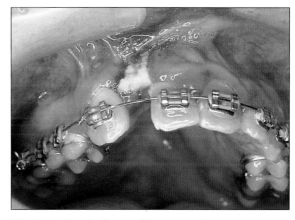

Fig 6-1 Cortical-cancellous one-piece autogenous bone graft to a cleft palate. Dehiscence and sequestration have led to loss of the graft.

priate bridging, and an inadequate amount of residual bone. The resultant bony maxillary bridge in the cleft area is insufficient to accommodate the subsequent eruption of permanent teeth. Block one-piece grafts, therefore, usually do not provide sufficient bone for tooth eruption. Additionally, the bone in the cleft area is inadequate to maintain the position of the arch after orthodontic expansion and presents insufficient bone for a titanium root-form implant.

By 1970, primarily as a result of the experience of the European surgeons, bone grafting of clefts had been abandoned in many surgical centers worldwide.

In 1970,[1,2] at the University of California at Los Angeles, we undertook a new approach to the bone grafting of clefts. This approach involved the use of particulate marrow and cancellous bone (PMCB) taken from the iliac crest. Initially, surgical grafting by this procedure was performed on patients when they reached the age of approximately 10 years. We have since adjusted the timing, so that grafting is performed when patients reach the age of 5 to 6 years, which we believe is the proper patient age for bone grafting.

Harvesting and Placement of the Graft

The surgical technique for harvesting the iliac crest bone graft in young children is similar to the procedure already described in chapter 1. The iliac bone is exposed inferior or dorsal to the crestal aponeurosis of the gluteus medius muscle, and a window in the lateral cortex for the harvesting of the bone is opened approximately 1.5 cm below the crest. There is no interference with the growth pattern of the ilium and no resultant osseous defect at the donor site. It is important, in this approach, to make the lateral table window inferior (or dorsal) to the apophysis. The epiphysis will regenerate with no residual osseous deficit and without any interference in growth of the ilium. A split crest technique can also be used if the surgeon desires, but the crest must be carefully reapproximated after the cancellous bone is harvested. If the crestal bone lateral or medial to the apophysis is lost, there will be a deficit and a resultant interference in iliac crest growth.

Figures 6-2a to 6-2d show placement of a PMCB graft in a young child and closure of the palatal mucosa as well as the labial soft-tissue flap to secure the soft tissue and obtain complete closure over the graft.

Long-term Results

Grafting

We have recently reported a long-term review of alveolar grafting comparing pregraft and postgraft arch expansion orthodontically.[2,3] In this case review, we wished to obtain additional information on the appropriate time for stimulation of the graft to determine if orthodontic tooth movement or transverse arch expansion would stimulate the graft and result in regeneration of a greater osseous mass of bone. The sequencing of the bone grafting of clefts and orthodontic treatment was found to be extremely important to the overall success of the grafting procedure.

In the follow-up evaluation of PMCB grafting in clefts of the maxilla we evaluated[2,3]:

1. The effectiveness of the closure of the soft-tissue oronasal fistula.
2. Improvement in skeletal relationships by cephalometric analysis using both frontal and profile views.
3. Overall esthetic considerations.
4. Occlusal relationships of the teeth, particularly the final erupted position of the canine in the area of the previous clefts.

Evaluation of the effect of appropriate stimulation of the graft postoperatively by arch expansion, tooth eruption, and normal growth was a principal objective of this study.

Long-term Results

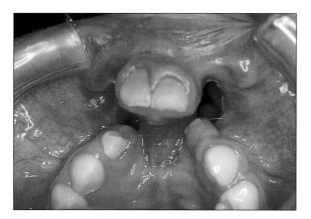

Fig 6-2a Maxillary cleft with a large osseous defect between the premaxilla and the maxilla.

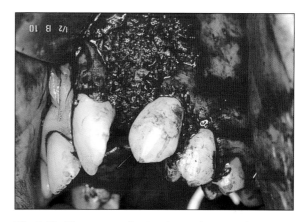

Fig 6-2b Placement of a PMCB graft.

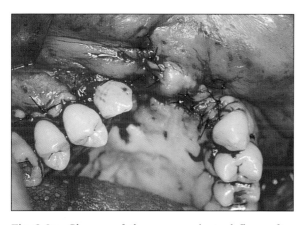

Fig 6-2c Closure of the mucoperiosteal flaps after grafting.

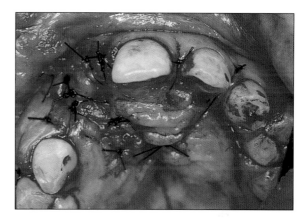

Fig 6-2d Closure of the palatal soft-tissue flap.

Postgrafting Arch Expansion

Most patients, particularly during the past 10 years, have been treated with the PMCB graft and postgrafting arch expansion. Orthodontic stimulation of the graft area is accomplished within 6 to 16 months after the grafting procedure.

In younger patients, in whom permanent teeth are not available, a completely soft-tissue–borne appliance is used for postgrafting arch expansion. When the 6-year molar is available, a palatal arch appliance is made to expand and stimulate the grafted area to reduce the patient's transverse posterior crossbite, which tends to occur in individuals with untreated cleft. Once this expansion is completed, the patient is monitored for the eruption of the teeth, particularly the canine tooth, which will erupt approximately 3 to 4 years

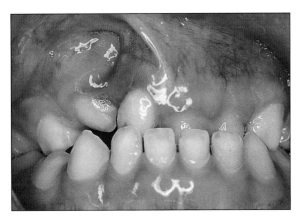

Fig 6-3 Unilateral cleft prior to bone grafting. The permanent central incisors are blocked lingually. Such an anterior crossbite requires correction immediately after bone grafting.

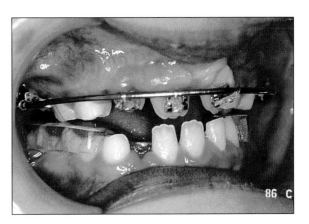

Fig 6-4 Orthopedic appliance opening the bite after grafting so that the central incisors can be "jumped" anteriorly into the proper position.

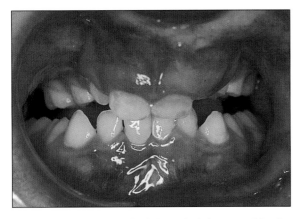

Fig 6-5 Similar case of a bilateral cleft, treated in the same manner as the cleft in Fig 6-4, shown approximately 1 year after grafting. The central incisors are in the correct position.

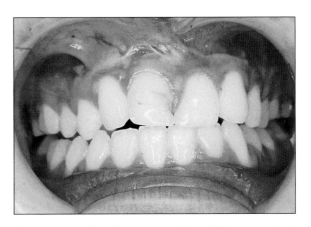

Fig 6-6 Completed treatment (in a different patient) is shown 5 years after grafting and after completion of orthodontic treatment.

after grafting. Using this protocol, we now graft patients when they reach the age of 5 to 6 years. A pre–bone-grafting view of a unilateral cleft (Fig 6-3) reveals that the maxillary incisor teeth are palatally displaced and "locked" lingually. After grafting is completed, an orthodontic appliance is used to move the maxillary incisors out of the anteroposterior crossbite (Fig 6-4). When the maxillary incisors are in the correct anteroposterior position, the growth of the maxilla is not inhibited (Fig 6-5). In another case, a bilateral cleft was treated in a similar manner, and the occlusion is excellent 5 years after grafting (Fig 6-6).

Long-term Results

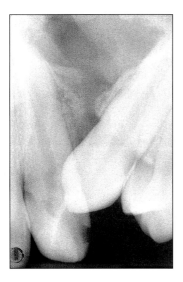
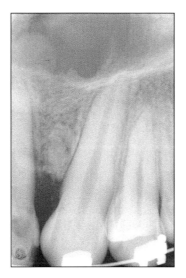
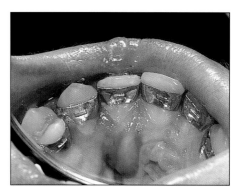

Fig 6-7a Eruption of the canine tooth into the area of the osseous defect in the cleft palate.

Fig 6-7b Postgrafting movement of the canine tooth to the central incisor to close the dental arch without leaving an edentulous space in the cleft area.

Fig 6-7c Completed eruption of the canine, which was brought adjacent to the central incisor. Maintenance of the crestal alveolar height is excellent when the clefts are treated with a combination of orthodontic treatment and bone grafting.

Alignment of Teeth

After PMCB grafting, the alignment of the teeth may be approached by one of two methods: by moving the canines medially to the position of the lateral incisor or by moving the canines laterally. When the canine tooth is moved adjacent to the central incisor orthodontically after grafting, the dental arch is completed without the necessity of prosthetic replacement (Figs 6-7a to 6-7c). When the canine is moved laterally to create an edentulous space, a prosthesis is required. Until recently, this has been a fixed partial denture on a removable appliance.

Moving the Canines Medially in the Cleft Area

Movement of canines adjacent to the central incisor after grafting has the following advantages: (1) The bone moves with the canine through the grafted area; (2) esthetics is improved; (3) there is less relapse of the premaxilla postoperatively; (4) eruption of the canine tooth into the grafted area stimulates bone formation and brings about an increase in the height and the width of the crest of the ridge; and (5) the need for a prosthesis is avoided. Figure 6-7c shows the erupted canine in the cleft area on the right; the alveolar bone has increased occlusally with the erupting tooth, resulting in an increase in alveolar ridge height. Excellent crestal bone is present both palatally and lingually.

Moving the Canines Laterally

Lateral movement of the canine after bone grafting creates an edentulous space in the cleft area. Until recently, these areas have been treated with fixed prostheses. However, patients have experienced a slow degeneration and resorption of the alveolar crest, as would be expected under any prosthetic appliance as the patient ages. Such cleft areas are now restored with root-form implant–borne prostheses to maintain the bone in the grafted area.

Timing of Grafting

Delaying bone grafting to the ages of 13 to 20 years decreases the ability to achieve orthodontic control of the premaxilla, leading to relapse. Patients now undergo the grafting procedure at the age of 5 to 6 years, and the central incisors are moved from their usual torqued position into the correct position within 1 year after grafting.

The result of a recent survey, in which patients were followed for 25 years postoperatively, supports the protocol for grafting at earlier ages (between 5 and 7 years) and reveals the importance of post–bone-grafting arch expansion. This protocol is therefore recommended as a most important part of the overall rehabilitation of these patients.

From a dental restorative standpoint, PMCB grafts establish the basis for early prosthodontic restoration of the cleft defect without interference in the normal growth patterns of the child. In addition, root-form titanium implants may be used in growing children.

Root-form Implants in Cleft Areas

Advantages

If the canine tooth has been moved laterally to create an edentulous space in the cleft area, we have been using, for the past 9 years, root-form titanium implants as a basis for prosthetic replacement. Since 1988, these implants have been very successful when placed with an augmentation graft of PMCB and Bio-Oss porous bone mineral (Geistlich Sons/ Osteohealth Co).

The root-form implants preserve the alveolar ridge height, stabilize the arch, and maintain the alveolar bone. The placement of titanium implants in the grafted cleft area prevents the long-term loss of bone from the alveolar ridge in the cleft area as the patient ages.

Placement Techniques

Bilateral and Unilateral Clefts

Implants are placed with the use of additional bone grafts, consisting of PMCB and Bio-Oss, in both the floor of the nose and in the crest area to increase ridge height in two important areas: the retrograde apical area (nasal floor) and the occlusal portion of the alveolar ridge (Fig 6-8a). This procedure increases the vertical height of the restored alveolar ridge, making possible use of longer implants, which add to the stability of the prosthesis.

The implants are placed into the thin alveolar bone bridge in a slightly labial position so that the apex is 2 to 3 mm into the nasal floor. The implants are loaded after 4 to 5 months with a fixed prosthesis. An older patient who is missing a lateral incisor in the area of the cleft and exhibits incomplete bony bridging of the area from a bone graft placed 5 years previ-

Placement Techniques

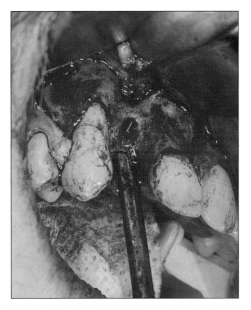

Fig 6-8a Cleft palate in which the canine has been moved laterally, producing room for a root-form implant. A root-form implant will be placed, and PMCB and Bio-Oss will be inserted in the occlusal portion as well as in the apical portion (the nasal floor).

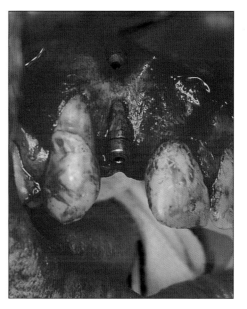

Fig 6-8b Placement of the implant.

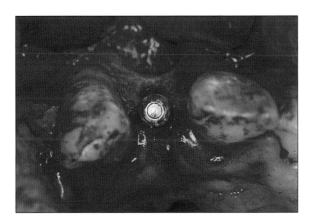

Fig 6-8c Lateral and palatal deficiencies, which also require grafting.

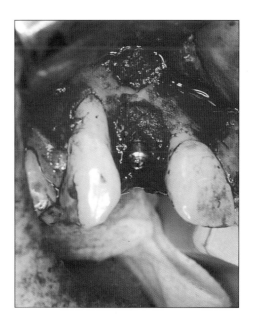

Fig 6-8d Placement of the implant with the final bone graft in the nasal floor and in the occlusal portion. Alveolar augmentation with the graft material makes possible the successful placement of implants in cleft areas of children and adults.

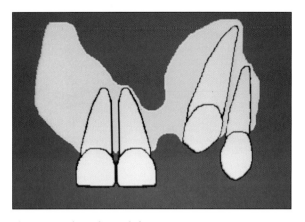

Fig 6-9a Edentulous cleft area.

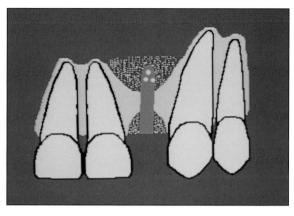

Fig 6-9b Graft and titanium implant in place.

ously is shown in Figs 6-8a to 6-8d. The augmentation PMCB and Bio-Oss graft can be seen in the floor of the nose and also increasing the ridge height inferiorly. These principles are illustrated in Figs 6-9a and 6-9b.

The bone graft may be maintained in height and width by using a titanium mesh (Ti-Mesh) implant (Figs 6-10a to 6-10c). The titanium mesh is removed after 3 months, and the prosthesis is completed. The placement of the abutments after 5 months is shown in Fig 6-10d, and the final fixed prosthesis with excellent function and esthetics is shown in Figs 6-10e and 6-10f.

Root-form implants may be placed in a grafted cleft when the patient reaches the age of 7 to 8 years. The titanium implant does not interfere with normal growth if it is placed correctly in the arch. The normal growth of the premaxilla is downward and forward and is both sutural and appositional. If the implants are placed slightly labially in the arch, there is no interference in growth or displacement of the prosthesis with the growth of the child.

Midline Clefts

The midline cleft is treated similarly to bilateral clefts: The PMCB graft is placed in the cleft defect, and the dentition is restored with root-form implants and a fixed implant-borne prosthesis. The same attention is given to the growth and development potential of the premaxilla. Some patients with long-standing bilateral clefts present with a completely atrophied premaxilla. These patients resemble those with a midline cleft. Such defects are treated in the same manner. Because midline clefts have no premaxillary bony segment, a bony floor of the anterior palate and premaxillary pyriform area must be established first by means of the TiMesh orthopedic implant (TiMesh, Inc) with PMCB and Bio-Oss grafts (Figs 6-11 to 6-13).

The initial bony defect is later augmented by a second TiMesh-supported bone graft of the same type of graft material. At the time of placement of the secondary graft, the root-form implant or implants are placed.

Placement Techniques

Figs 6-10a to 6-10f Use of titanium mesh in the cleft palate of an adult patient.

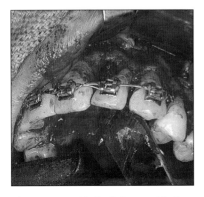

Fig 6-10a Cleft defect with impending loss of the lateral and central incisors on the cleft side.

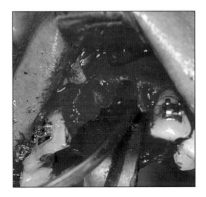

Fig 6-10b Osseous defect showing a small, incomplete bridge of bone prior to grafting.

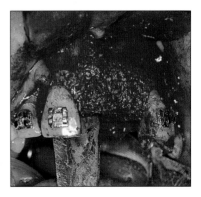

Fig 6-10c Placement of the graft (PMCB and Bio-Oss).

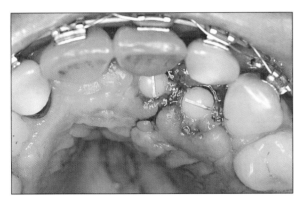

Fig 6-10d Healing abutments, placed 5 months after implant integration. (Implants were placed 4 months after bone grafting.) Provisional crowns are attached to the orthodontic arch bar.

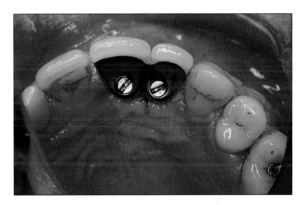

Fig 6-10e Completed prosthesis. Maintenance of alveolar ridge height and width is excellent.

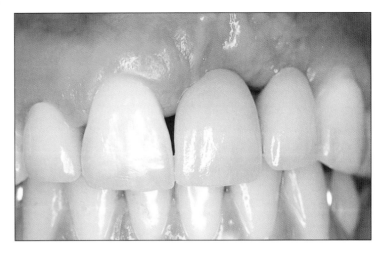

Fig 6-10f Clinical view of the prosthesis.

83

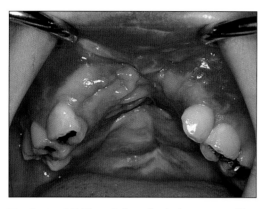

Fig 6-11a Midline cleft and missing premaxilla.

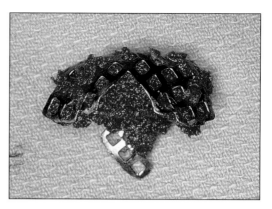

Fig 6-11b Titanium mesh filled with PMCB and Bio-Oss graft material.

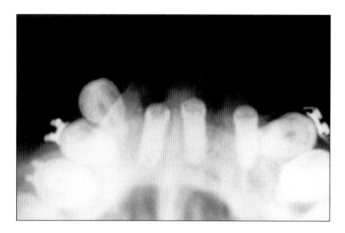

Fig 6-11c Final osseous ridge with implants in place. The implants were placed 5 months after grafting.

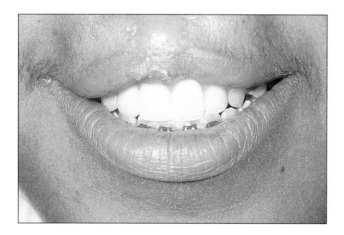

Fig 6-12 Completed prosthesis.

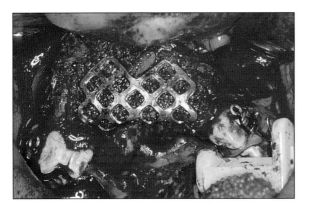

Fig 6-13a Large midline cleft being restored with the titanium mesh in a procedure similar to that shown in Figs 6-11 and 6-12.

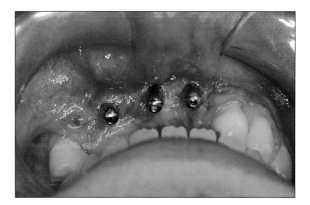

Fig 6-13b Abutments placed 5 months after implant placement, which was accomplished at the time of removal of the TiMesh.

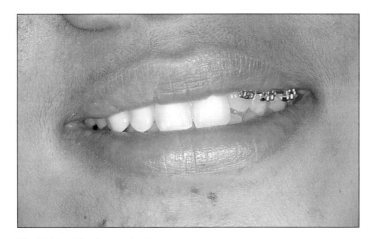

Fig 6-13c Final prosthesis.

In summary, with the use of PMCB grafting, the reconstruction of unilateral, bilateral, and midline clefts has been made possible, allowing prosthodontic restoration with excellent and predictable functional and esthetic results. This sequenced surgical grafting procedure has been very successful in restoring large unilateral or bilateral clefts of the maxilla. A 5-year–postoperative review of patients treated in this manner indicated that the extent of the osseous restoration (width and height) is clinically and radiographically maintained. This maintenance of the osseous alveolar ridge and the anterior part of the maxilla results from the type of graft used (composite autograft and xenogeneic porous bone mineral) and the presence of the root-form implants in the restored ridge.

References

1. Boyne PJ. Use of marrow cancellous bone grafts in maxillary alveolar and palatal clefts. J Dent Res 1974;43:821–824.
2. Boyne PJ. Bone grafting in the osseous reconstruction of alveolar and palatal clefts. Oral Maxillofac Surg Clin North Am 1991;3:589–597.
3. Boyne PJ, Scheer PM. Long-term study of autogenously bone grafted bilateral alveolar clefts. In: Pfeifer G (ed). Proceedings of the 4th Hamburg International Symposium on Craniofacial Anomalies and Clefts of Lip, Alveolus, and Palate. Stuttgart: Thieme, 1991:349–355.

Characterization of Xenogeneic Bone Material

Michael Peetz

Both autogenous bone grafts (from the patient's own body) and allogeneic (or homologous) banked bone (from another individual of the same species) are frequently and successfully employed to promote regeneration of parts of the skeleton. The use of these types of grafts is limited, however, by the cost of a donor site operation for autogenous bone or by fear of the risk of infection (with human immunodeficiency virus, hepatitis, etc) with use of allogeneic materials. Limited end results have been produced by alloplastic materials (synthetic bone substitutes).

A fourth type of graft uses xenogeneic material (bone taken from another species, ie, animal bone). Until recently, this type of graft was not employed, because of possible immunologic response to the organic portion of the material. This appendix describes the development of a totally biocompatible xenogeneic porous bone mineral that possesses many properties of an ideal bone substitute.

Characterization of Bone Graft Substitutes

Characterization and analysis of any bone graft substitute prior to its use in human bone sites involves consideration of several material properties of the graft:

1. Chemical and physiologic composition
2. Morphologic structure
3. Physical properties
4. Absence of xenogeneic, allogeneic, and/or other foreign protein in the material

Based on these properties, ideal bone substitutes should demonstrate:

1. Excellent biocompatibility, to be fully accepted by the living organism.
2. High osteoconductivity, to promote conduction of new bone formation from the walls of the host bone defect.
3. A large inner surface area, to become fully revascularized by the host bone site.
4. High porosity, to be completely incorporated in new bone.

5. Moderately slow resorption, to remain in place, promoting long-term bone remodeling.
6. An adequate modulus of elasticity, to guarantee a natural stress/strain environment.

Characterization of Natural Bone Mineral (Bio-Oss)

When the organic material is removed from xenogeneic bone, a special mild treatment must be used to preserve the original composition and structure of the inorganic substance. The technical process used in producing the xenograft Bio-Oss (Geistlich Sons/ Osteohealth Co) from a bovine bone source makes possible the removal of all organic components of the bone product, leaving a pure, nonorganic bone matrix in unchanged inorganic form. Bio-Oss is a finely crystalline, carbonated apatite practically identical to natural human bone mineral. The chemical extraction process makes possible the desirable properties of this material.

The implantation of Bio-Oss in surgical sites leads to ample formation of well-vascularized new bone, which integrates with the Bio-Oss particles to restore proper structure and function in the defect site. The resulting high bone-to-matrix ratio gives the surgeon an excellent basis for operations involving use of titanium root-form implants or orthopedic devices in reconstructive or orthognathic surgery.

Chemical and Physical Composition

Chemical Composition

The chemical composition of Bio-Oss has been extensively analyzed by infrared spectrometry. The infrared spectrum (Fig A-1) shows that synthetic hydroxyapatites have more nanomeric hydroxyl groups than does natural bone or Bio-Oss.[1]

Bio-Oss retains the natural mineral content of bone, which has a more complex composition than do synthetic hydroxyapatites. The chemical composition of a graft material influences the rate and extent to which it is incorporated into the host tissue and the subsequent physical characteristics of the graft site.

Crystalline Structure

Even more important is the crystalline structure of biomaterials. Bio-Oss bone consists of very tiny crystals similar to those of human bone. The small crystals are represented in x-ray diffraction analysis by broad interference lines, resulting in a very broad spectrum. The huge crystals of synthetic materials, on the other hand, represent small interference lines and show a characteristically narrow spectrum.

Differences in the major bone substitute materials currently being marketed are even more apparent when the crystalline structures of bone and various bone graft substitutes are compared by transmission electron microscopy.[2] The measurements shown for natural bone mineral (Bio-Oss) are characteristic of the tiny crystal size observed in normal human bone (Table A-1).

Small crystals present a very large surface area. In general, bone material is very sensitive to any kind of energy. One method of removing the organic material is by heating. However, when crystals are heated to temperatures of about 600°C, recrystallization takes place, the crystals tend to grow, and the structure of the material changes. At the same time 4.8% of the constituents are lost, and the composition is modified. As a result, the overall surface shrinks, the "pores" tend to be lost, and the elasticity is reduced.

Characterization of Natural Bone Mineral (Bio-Oss)

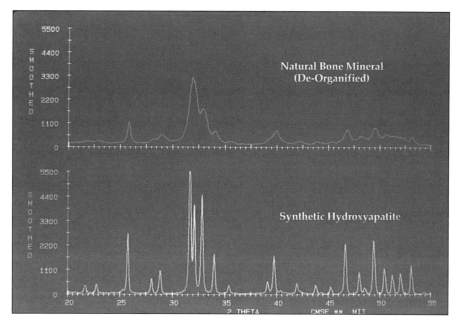

Fig A-1 X-ray diffraction analysis comparing the inorganic structures of Bio-Oss and synthetic hydroxyapatite.

Table A-1 Comparison of bone graft substitutes by transmission electron microscopy*

Material	Supplier	Particle size† (nm)	Particle shape
Human cancellous bone chips	Pacific Coast Tissue Bank	10–50	Thin and tiny elongated platelets in a fibrous matix
Bio-Oss	Geistlich and Sons Wolhusen, Switzerland	10–60	Thin and tiny platelets, fairly homogenous in size and shape
Osteograft/N	CeraMed Lakewood, CO	1000–5000 100,000	Inhomogenous: larger particles and coarse grains
OsteoGen	Impladent Hollisville, NY	500–5000 and >100,000	Heterogenous: smaller platelets and druses
Interpore 200	Interpore International Irving, CA	100–1000	Platelets with a broad distribution of particle sizes

* Results obtained by Prof Dr Rudolf Giovanoli, Laboratory for Electron Microscopy, University of Bern, Bern, Switzerland.

† The size of these particles could be estimated from the width of the interferences in the x-ray diffractograms using the equation of Debye-Scherrer. The size of Bio-Oss crystals was found to be similar, within the confidence limits, of the size of human natural bone particles. All other products showed crystal structures larger than those of natural bone.

Unlike this heat treatment, the mild treatment used in the preparation of Bio-Oss preserves the original composition and structure of the crystals. The crystal structures of the hydroxyapatites in bone products treated with high temperatures (eg, Osteograft/N) exhibit crystalline enlargement. The result is huge crystals, which form a dense and a very stiff material unlike the flexible bone structure of natural bone mineral (Bio-Oss).

The biologic effect of crystal growth in bone products was also reported by Jensen et al,[1] who measured a significantly higher degree of osseointegration after 8 weeks with Bio-Oss than with a bone-derived material obtained by using temperatures greater than 1,000°C.

Morphologic Structure

Porosity

The spongiosa structure shown in Fig A-2 demonstrates the wide interconnective pore system of natural bone mineral. These pores can easily be invaded by new blood vessels, which is followed by osteoblastic migration. Natural bone mineral (Bio-Oss) consists of the following porosity systems:

1. Macropores: pores in a visible range of 300 to 1,500 µm (Fig A-2)
2. Micropores: typical haversian canals and smaller vascular marrow channels in the bone structure (Fig A-3)
3. Intercrystalline spaces: small pores in the range of 3 to 26 nm (Fig A-4).

These pore systems result in an overall porosity of 70% to 75%. When material such as Bio-Oss natural bone mineral is placed into a given defect, it usually occupies only 25% to 30% of the defect, leaving 75% of the space for regeneration of new bone tissue. No other currently available synthetic material reaches these high porosity numbers. This surface condition enhances the penetration of host bone repair into the inner part of the graft material.

Surface

In addition to the porosity of bone substitute materials, the inner surface must be considered. Measurements by mercury porosimetry have shown that most existing synthetic hydroxyapatites have a specific surface of approximately 1 to 10 m^2/g (Table A-2). Table A-2 presents the results of the measurement for various hydroxyapatites and human bone. Only Osteogen represents a higher surface with 26.9 m^2. However, this material consists of inhomogenous crystal structures with smaller platelets and large druses. Bio-Oss, on the other hand, presents an homogenous crystalline structure (see Fig A-3).

As shown in Table A-2, Bio-Oss reaches a surface of almost 100 m^2/g. This huge surface allows it to achieve intimate contact with osteoblasts and pluripotential osteogenic cells. With such a pore system, Bio-Oss may easily be penetrated and invaded by bone-forming cells of the host. Figure A-4 shows the complex surface of Bio-Oss. This complex type of surface has not been replicated by a synthetic material produced in the laboratory. Osteoblasts "recognize" the Bio-Oss surfaces, which consist of biologic apatite as a bone layer, and these cells use that surface for deposition of new bone.

Physical Properties

The physical properties of Bio-Oss have been investigated by Myron Spector[3] of Harvard University. Measurements were taken to define the compressive strength and modulus of elasticity of this material. Spector's work makes clear that any material implanted in

Characterization of Natural Bone Mineral (Bio-Oss)

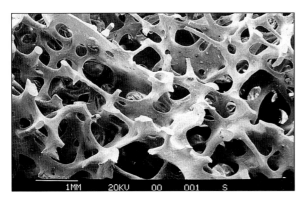

Fig A-2 Scanning electron micrograph of Bio-Oss cancellous structure. (Original magnification ×40.)

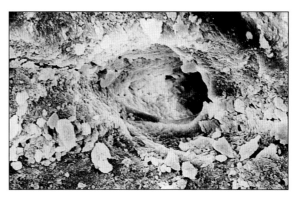

Fig A-3 Scanning electron micrograph of an opening of a haversian canal. (Original magnification ×1000.)

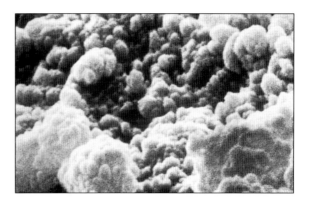

Fig A-4 Scanning electron micrograph of the surface of a Bio-Oss particle. (Original magnification ×100,000.)

Table A-2 Comparison of bone graft substitutes by mercury porosimetry*†

Material	Inner surface (%)	Inner surface‡ (m^2/g)	More frequent pore size (nm)
Human cancellous bone chips	7.1	1.4 (filled with protein)	—
Bio-Oss	60.0	97.0	23
Osteograft/N	29.4	1.0	195
OsteoGen	60.3	26.9	13 and 65
Interpore 200	16.4	3.1	35

* Measurements performed by Dr Günther Kahr, Institute for Geotechnic, Swiss Federal Institute of Technology, Zurich, Switzerland.

† The measurements were made at pressures up to 4,000 bar.

‡ The mineral of the human cancellous bone will have a porosity and inner surface at least equal to those of Bio-Oss. However, these measurements cannot reveal it: the interstitial spaces of the one are occupied by collagen and dead protein. Mercury, therefore, cannot enter the pore system. With the other products also containing no collagen, the effectively smaller inner surface as a result of the rigorous treatment is measured.

Table A-3 Mechanical properties of bone graft substitutes*

Material	Compressive strength (MPa)	Modulus of elasticity (GPa)
Cortical bone	140	14
Cancellous bone	5–60	1.4
Anorganic bone (Bio-Oss) cortical	35	11
Synthetic hydroxyapatite (Calcitek)	200–900	34–100

* From Spector.[1]

Absence of Protein

Absence of any protein in the bone substrate material is important to be certain that no allergic or immunologic reaction occurs after implantation of the xenograft material in human patients. The complete removal of all organic materials is confirmed for each batch of Bio-Oss material produced.

Three different chemical methods are applied to demonstrate the complete absence of protein. Total protein is measured by the method described by Lowry et al[4] with a detection limit of 135 ppm. Collagen components are measured by detection of any 4-hydroxyproline with a detection limit of 23 ppm. Amino acids and amines are measured down to a detection limit of 4 ppm.[5]

Cohen et al[6] assessed the potential inflammatory changes associated with Bio-Oss and Bio-Oss collagen. Histologic examination of specimens after the implantation of these materials into soft tissue and bone revealed no signs of inflammation. Between 3 days and 8 weeks after subcutaneous placement in the dorsal skin sites of rats, sites were evaluated. Administration of saline alone and mineral oil served as negative and positive controls, respectively. Hydroxyapatite (Interpore 200 granules and block) was used as a treatment control. For identification of inflammatory reactions, a panel of six different monoclonal antibodies was used. There was no increase in monocytes, tissue macrophages, lymphoid macrophages, 1a antigens, T and B lymphocytes, or various monoclonal antibodies in Bio-Oss treated sites. A slight infiltration with macrophages was observed with all grafts. This infiltrate returned to a physiologic level at 3 days. Neither a local nor a general systemic inflammatory reaction appeared after Bio-Oss implantation. The results were consistent with those found for synthetic hydroxyapatite grafting materials.

bone tissue should have characteristics similar to those of the surrounding host bone, to avoid microfractures at the graft–host bone interface.

The measurements by Spector[3] show that the compressive strengths of Bio-Oss and bone are in the same range (Table A-3). The compressive strength represents the power that has to be applied to a material to compress it and shatter the specimen. The synthetic hydroxyapatites show compressive strengths of 200 to 900 MPa. That represents a higher stiffness and a higher density for synthetic materials in comparison to surrounding host recipient bone. Such a high density tends to produce problems at the implanted material–host bone interface.

These characteristics result in a higher modulus of elasticity. Measurements were 14 GPa for cortical bone and 11 GPa for the anorganic xenograft bone Bio-Oss, representing approximately the same elasticity for bone and Bio-Oss (see Table A-3). Synthetic hydroxyapatites, on the other hand, show values of 35 to 100 GPa. This higher stiffness and lower flexibility may, under long-term function, cause stress at the interface. Resulting microfractures between graft and host bone can lead to fibrous encapsulation of synthetic bone substitutes.

The absence of antigenic response from the porous bone mineral was also proven with enzyme-linked immunosorbent assay in a rabbit model with implantation times between 4 weeks and 6 months in the femoral bone.[7] The histologic investigation over 1 year in rabbits and rats revealed no evidence of neoplastic change and no atypical cytoplasmic or nuclear structures. Clinical long-term studies[8] and over 12 to 16 months in monkeys[9] also failed to indicate any abnormal cellular reactions.

In summary, investigations have shown Bio-Oss to have a natural morphologic structure; a chemical composition identical to that of bone; a large inner surface and porosity comparable to that of bone; a crystalline structure identical to that of bone tissue; and a composition that is purely anorganic.

Biologic Characteristics (Product Design)

Before bone graft substitutes can be used effectively, certain questions have to be answered. First, the degree of host bone incorporation of the biomaterial must be known. For example, is an extensive chemical bone binding achieved or does bone repair occur secondarily by contact with the host bone cells? Second, the question of resorption of the surrounding bone and of the material itself must be investigated. Are the bone and the graft allowed to achieve physiologic remodeling? Third, the question of load support is important for long-term results. Fourth, the ability of a material to be drilled into, producing an osteotomy for the implantation of titanium fixtures, must be determined.

Bone Formation

The biologic character of Bio-Oss has been examined in a number of animal and clinical experiments (Table A-4). The bone formation process has been studied by Schlickewei.[10] Bio-Oss implanted in the rabbit femoral bone was analyzed over an observation period of 1 year. Analysis after 1 month, 6 months, and 12 months showed that the new bone contact of the Bio-Oss surface is enhanced with time. After 1 year, 90.83% of the Bio-Oss surface is covered by new bone (Figs A-5 and A-6).

Table A-4 Animal and clinical experiments used to assess the biologic characteristics of Bio-Oss

Implantation Site	Method of outcome measurement
Soft tissue	Histology
Femur	Histomorphometric evaluation
Tibia	Polychrome markers
Mandible/maxilla	Radiograph
Calvarium	ELISA test (antigenicity)
Iliac crest	Antibody trapping
Control group osseous sites	Biomechanics

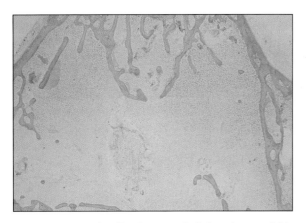

Fig A-5 Standardized control defect in a rabbit femur, showing lack of filling with repair bone after 6 months. (Histologic specimen; courtesy of Prof R. Schenk, University of Bern, Bern, Switzerland.)

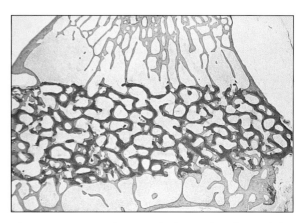

Fig A-6 Bone matrix around Bio-Oss in a femoral defect of a rabbit, showing regeneration after 6 months. New cortical surface has formed from remodeling of the area.

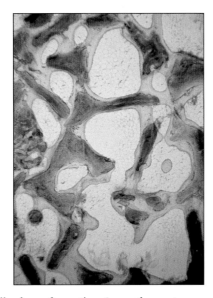

Fig A-7 Lamellar bone formation 6 months postoperatively, showing integration of the Bio-Oss matrix in the repair bone of the defect. (Original magnification ×16). (Histologic specimen; courtesy of Prof R. Schenk, University of Bern.)

Histomorphometric analysis over the 1-year period showed that the quantity of Bio-Oss decreases slightly over time, while new bone quantity increases. After 12 months, approximately the same amounts of Bio-Oss and new bone are seen, representing 60% of the complete bone tissue. The remaining area (40%) is filled by bone marrow. This compares favorably with normal bone tissue structure (Fig A-7).

Boyne[11] demonstrated an enhancement of total bone matrix in the diaphysis of the femur of rhesus monkeys after implantation of porous Bio-Oss. The study was done to determine if porous bone mineral could be used to increase bone density in femoral shafts scheduled for press-fitted implants as part of a total hip prosthesis study. The work indicated that, as bone is slowly remodeled, the surgical area takes on an increased bone matrix density that is sustained for a prolonged period, thus indicating the possibility of using Bio-Oss in areas of decreased bone density (eg, femoral shafts and the posterior maxilla) to enhance the recipient bone's ability to sustain implantation of metal.

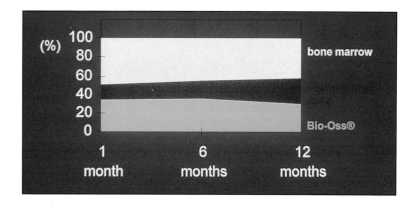

Fig A-8 Histomorphometric results of analysis of bone regeneration with Bio-Oss spongiosa after 12 months.

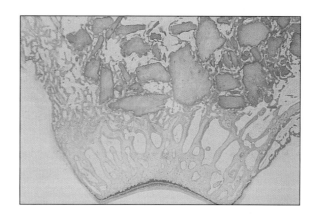

Fig A-9 Regeneration of a femoral defect in a rabbit with Bio-Oss corticalis. (Histologic specimen; courtesy of Prof R. Schenk, University of Bern.)

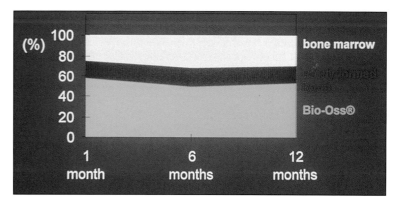

Fig A-10 Histomorphometric results of bone regeneration with Bio-Oss corticalis after 12 months.

The analysis of implanted Bio-Oss cancellous granules and Bio-Oss cancellous block did not reveal significant differences between the two types (Fig A-8).

To distinguish the qualitative and quantitative differences of cortical and cancellous Bio-Oss, cortical particles were also implanted in the femoral bones of rabbits (Fig A-9). Measurements over 12 months showed that the implantation of Bio-Oss cortical particles represented a filling by Bio-Oss and new bone of approximately 50% of the defect structure (Fig A-10), while the Bio-Oss spongiosa filled up approximately 33% of the defect after implantation. Consequently, the Bio-Oss spongiosa offers greater space for the regeneration

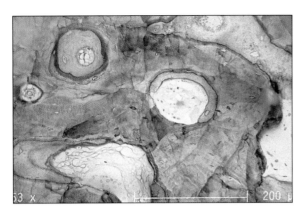 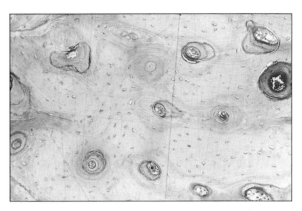

Fig A-11 Revascularization of a Bio-Oss particle. The osteons of the Bio-Oss particles are invaded by new bone with accompanying angiogenesis. (Histologic specimen; courtesy of Prof Schenk, University of Bern.)

Fig A-12 New bone and blood vessels have invaded the "interporosity" areas of a Bio-Oss particle from a human biopsy specimen at 8 months. (Histologic specimen; courtesy of Prof R Schenk, University of Bern.)

of new bone tissue and seems to be the material of choice for the regenerative process in the maxilla and the mandible. The enlargement of the histologic views showed, for both Bio-Oss spongiosa and Bio-Oss cortical bone, internal pores that are filled by new bone. Porous areas with diameters of approximately 80 μm and more were invaded by new bone (Fig A-11).

To distinguish between the blood vessels from Bio-Oss and those from newly formed bone, Schenk[12] used a different staining method. The number of blood vessels penetrating a Bio-Oss cortical particle was impressive and demonstrated the revascularizing and remodeling of the anorganic material through the invasion of blood vessels and new bone (Fig A-12).

Spector[3] implanted Bio-Oss in 30 rabbits and evaluated the results after 10, 20, and 40 days. As a control, synthetic calcium phosphate was used. These results were evaluated by histomorphometric methods. Figure A-13 shows a defect that has been filled with the synthetic material. The structure of the material varies significantly from the surrounding bone spongious structure.

In contrast, 1 week after implantation of Bio-Oss, osteoblasts are lining up and starting the mineralization process to form new matrix. A line of osteoid tends to form, embedding the osteoblastic cells in the mineral matrix. The osteoid covers the Bio-Oss surfaces and represents the first immature bone. This bone formation continues and will lead to the union of bone matrix and Bio-Oss particles across the defect to the walls of the host defect (Fig A-14).

Six weeks after implantation, the newly formed bone is interconnecting the Bio-Oss particles (Fig A-15). The bridging by new bone is leading to the stabilization of the host bone in the defect area. Figure A-16 presents an overview of the healed area and the new bone repair structure that has been built with the help of Bio-Oss. The particles are difficult to recognize and distinguish from the surrounding bone tissue because of the intense proliferation of new osseous repair matrix.

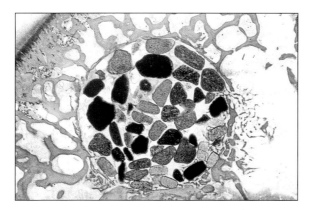

Fig A-13 Medial condyle of a rabbit. Overall view of the surgical defect 40 days after use of a synthetic hydroxyapatite structure, revealing a demarcation between the nonporous hydroxyapatite and the host bone matrix. There is a lack of bone formation around the individual particles of hydroxyapatite.

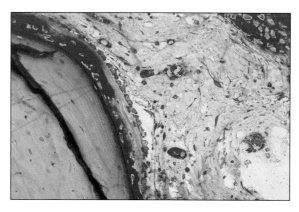

Fig A-14 Osteoid building on the surface of a particle of Bio-Oss. New osteoblasts are overlying the mineralized matrix on the Bio-Oss surface. (Histologic specimen; courtesy of Dr M. Spector, Boston.)

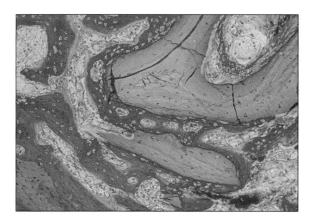

Fig A-15 Newly formed bone (dark staining) at 40 days, bridging over Bio-Oss particles in a rabbit femur defect. (Histologic specimen; courtesy of Dr M. Spector, Boston.)

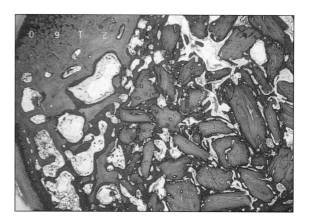

Fig A-16 Overall view of bone formation around Bio-Oss particles from a rabbit defect at 40 days. (Histologic specimen; courtesy of Dr M. Spector, Boston.)

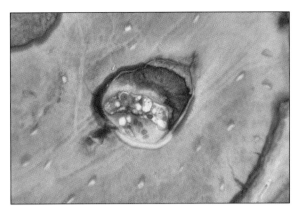

Fig A-17 Osteoclastic activity in the internal porosity area of a Bio-Oss particle adjacent to areas of bone formation from a human biopsy specimen (Prof R. Schenk, University of Bern.)

Bone Remodeling

Indications of the resorption process can be identified by osteoclasts on the Bio-Oss surface next to areas of bone formation (Fig A-17). Bone is a living tissue that usually is transformed by approximately 2% to 3% per year by a constant remodeling process. In surgical defects, however, the bone may remodel faster from the woven bone, and the transforming process to lamellar bone may occur completely within several months, depending on various factors involving graft site, vascularity, and functional forces.

The remodeling process was studied in the femoral bone of rabbits after implantation of Bio-Oss in comparison with a synthetic hydroxyapatite. Kita et al[13] measured the number of osteoclasts on the new interstitial bone between the particles, on the particles themselves, and on the surface of the bone that surrounded the standardized defect. Their evaluation clearly showed that more resorbing cells are present when Bio-Oss is implanted than when synthetic hydroxyapatite material is implanted in the same type of surgical defect (Fig A-18).

In addition, a higher number of osteoclast-like cells were observed on the surface of the interstitial bone that was connecting the particles. However, outside the defect, no difference in resorbing cells was seen whether Bio-Oss or the synthetic product was implanted. The results of this study[13] indicate that there may be an ongoing resorbing process when Bio-Oss is implanted. This is confirmed by the measurement of the Bio-Oss surface area, which declined over a period of 6 weeks. Table A-5 shows the changes in natural bone mineral (Bio-Oss) with time. Surface reduction of Bio-Oss after 10, 20, and 40 days is indicated by a decrease in the mean perimeter. The mean perimeter of the synthetic hydroxyapatite remains stable, indicating lack of remodeling.

The authors[13] emphasized the direct bonding of host bone to the Bio-Oss surface. According to Spector,[3] the natural bone mineral initially supplies the biologic apatite that is required for early bone formation through deposition of apatite crystals for the mineralization process.[14] This may also explain why the osteoconductive performance of Bio-Oss was much greater than that of synthetic hydroxyapatites.[1,15]

Resorption lacunae were also reported in human histologic specimens examined by Schenk.[12] Figures A-19a and A-19b show a drill cylinder taken 8 months after localized mandibular ridge augmentation with Bio-Oss and Bio-Gide (a resorbable bilayer membrane formed from collagen fibers; Geistlich Sons/Osteohealth Co). The cylinder shows reconstruction of the cortical crest with underlying spongiosa structures. Bio-Oss is integrated in the newly formed lamellar bone. Figure A-19b shows resorption lacunae in the specimen shown in Fig A-19a. The lacunae in the Bio-Oss particles are filled with new bone next to osteoclasts, indicating an ongoing remodeling process.

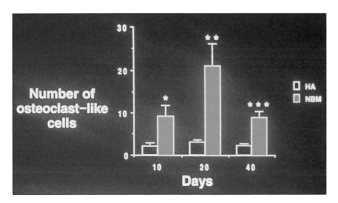

Fig A-18 Results of the study by Kita et al[13] indicating the number of osteoblasts on the surfaces of the particles.

Table A-5 Changes in Bio-Oss and synthetic hydroxyapatite (SHA) with time*

Time (d)	Mean perimeter (μm)	
	Bio-Oss	SHA
10	124	94
20	113	89
40	97	89

* These data were generated in a rabbit study, and it is known that rabbits have a much faster bone conversion process than do humans. A direct conversion of these data to humans has to be regarded with caution. Disagreement prevails on the biodegradation of Bio-Oss. Kita et al[13] reported a significant resorption of Bio-Oss and Klinge et al[15] found almost total resorption, Schlickewei and Paul[7] saw biodegradation to a lesser degree that could be described as physiologic remodeling.

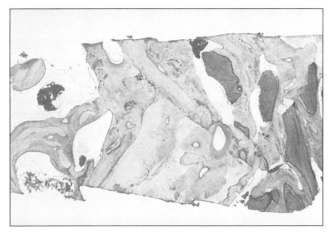

Fig A-19a Alveolar ridge reconstruction with Bio-Oss and Bio-Gide. Human specimen showing bone formation around particles at 8 months. (Histologic specimen; courtesy of Prof R. Schenk, University of Bern.)

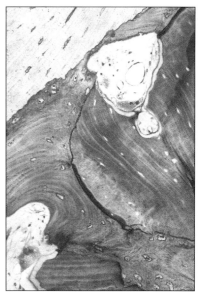

Fig A-19b Higher magnification of the specimen shown in Fig A-19a, revealing resorption. There are osteoblasts on the surface of a Bio-Oss particle, which is exhibiting ongoing resorption and remodeling.

These data indicate that the resorbing remodeling process may go on for years. This has also been confirmed in various investigations of human material. The initial integration of Bio-Oss into lamellar structures can be seen in the specimens. Later the resorbing process follows, involving the surrounding bone in a delayed remodeling processes. The normal osseous resorbing and remodeling rate occurring in functional cortical bone matrix is only between 2% and 3% per year, indicating that only a slow resorption of a material should occur after functional new bone structure has been established. Natural bone mineral displays a similar physiologic mechanism. This resorption, remodeling and new bone formation process is prolonged by the presence of residual Bio-Oss particles,[16] thus assuring a constant bone matrix density, an increase in bone density, and an increase of the thickness and quantity of osseous trabeculae and bone cortex. Boyne[9,16-17] has shown that the slow resorption and remodeling of porous bone mineral imparts a high degree of permanency to the restored mandibular edentulous area.

The physical and chemical properties of porous bone mineral (Bio-Oss) are host compatible, offering excellent conductive surfaces for the promotion of bone repair.

References

1. Jensen SS, Pinholt EM, Hjørting-Hansen E, Melsen F, Ruyter E. Tissue reaction and material characteristics of four bone substitutes. Int J Oral Maxillofac Implants (in press).
2. Giovanoli R. Laboratory for electron-microscopy. Project report, University of Bern, Switzerland, 8 Nov 1994.
3. Spector M. Anorganic bovine bone and ceramic analogs of bone mineral as implants to facilitate bone regeneration. Clin Plast Surg 1994;21:437–444.
4. Lowry OH, Rosebrough NJ, Farr AL, Randall RJ. Protein measurement with the folin phenol reagent. J Biol Chem 1951;193:265–275.
5. Al-Ghabsha TS, Rahim SA. Spectrophotometric determination of microgram amounts of amines with chloranil. Anal Chim Acta 1976;85:189–194.
6. Cohen RE, Mullarky RH, Noble B, Comeau RL, Nieders ME. Phenotypic characterization of mononuclear cells following anorganic bovine bone implantation in rats. J Periodontol 1994;65:1008–1015.
7. Schlickewei W, Paul C. Experimental investigations on bone replacement using bovine apatite. Unfallheilkunde 1991;216:59–69.
8. Boyne PJ. Vergleich von Bio-Oss und anderen Implantationsmaterialien bei der Erhaltung des Alveolarkammes des Unterkiefers beim Menschen. Unfallheilkunde 1991;216:98–103.
9. Boyne PJ. Host response to intraosseous implants placed in HA grafted mandibles. Mater Res Soc (Symp Proc) 1989;110:219–227.
10. Schlickewei W. Knochenersatz mit bovinem Apatit [thesis]. University of Freiburg, Germany, 1994.
11. Boyne PJ. Use of porous bone mineral to increase bone density. In: Pfeifer G (ed). [Proceedings of the Material Research Society Fall 1993 Symposium, Boston.] Material Research Symposium Proceedings 1993;331:263–265.
12. Schenk R. Berict über die histologische Untersuchung von 16 Biopsien nach oralchirurgischen Operationen mit Bio-Oss. Project report, Pathophysiology Institute, University of Bern, Switzerland, 5 Apr 1994.
13. Kita K, Rivin JM, Spector M. A Quantitative Characterization of the Osseous Response to Natural Bone Mineral and Synthetic Hydroxyapatite Ceramic. Boston: Harvard Medical School, 1991.
14. Peetz M. Properties of biomaterials for bone regeneration. In: Proceedings of the Giornate Internazionali di Implantologia Orale. Bologna, Italy: Monduzzi, 1994.
15. Klinge B, Alberius P, Isaksson S, Jönsson J. Osseous response to implanted natural bone mineral and synthetic hydroxylapatite ceramic in repair of experimental skull bone defects. J Oral Maxillofac Surg 1992;50:241–249.
16. Boyne PJ, Burnham M, Devlin M. Effect on bone morphology and alveolar contour of the socket in implantation of hydroxylapatite. Presented at the 4th International Congress in Preprosthetic Surgery, Palm Springs, CA, 18–20 Apr 1991.
17. Boyne PJ. Comparison of porous and nonporous hydroxyapatite and anorganic xenografts in the restoration of alveolar ridges. In: Proceedings of Symposium of the American Society for Testing and Materials. 1988:359–369.

Index

Page numbers followed by "f" indicate figures; numbers followed by "t" indicate tables.

A

Allogeneic grafts, 3, 87
Alloplastic materials, 3, 87
Alveolar ridge, PMCB and Bio-Oss in restoration of, 56, 57f
Antigeneic response, to Bio-Oss, 92–93
Arch expansion
  following PMCB grafting in cleft palate, 77–78, 78f
Atrophy
  mandibular
    PMCB and Bio-Oss graft, treatment with, 56, 57f
  maxillary
    titanium mesh in reconstruction following, 68f, 69
Autografts. *See* Autogenous grafts.
Autogenous grafts, 3, 87

B

Bar
  mandibular
    with IMZ implants, 58, 62f
    in oncologic surgical defect, 67f
    in prosthesis support, 50f
    on root-form implants, 45f
Bio-Oss (natural bone mineral)
  absence of protein in
    enzyme-linked immunosorbent assay for, 93
    histologic examination for, 92
  as barrier to ingrowth of connective tissue, 63–64, 64f
  biologic characteristics of
    in animal and clinical experiments, 93t
    bone formation and, 93–97
    bone remodeling and, 98, 98f, 99f, 100
  bone density increase with
    Macaca monkey study, 54, 55f
    Rhesus monkey study, 51f, 54
  as bone morphogenetic protein carrier, 15f, 18
  chemical composition of, 88, 89f
    comparison with synthetic hydroxypapatites, 89f
  comparison of spongiosa and corticalis
    in bone regeneration with, 95, 95f, 96f
  comparison with hydroxyapatite
    synthetic, 89f
  in conduction, 14f
  crystalline structure of, 88, 89t, 90
    comparison with other bone graft substitutes, 89t
  mechanical properties of, 92, 92t
  morphologic structure of
    comparison with other bone graft substitutes, 91t
    inner surface of, 90, 91f, 91t
    porosity systems of, 90, 91f
  physical properties of, 90, 92, 92f
    comparison with other substitutes, 92t
    compressive strength of, 92, 92t
    modulus of elasticity of, 92, 92t
BMP. *See* Bone morphogenetic protein (BMP).
Bone
  demineralized freeze-dried, 17
  density increase of, at titanium surface, 54, 56, 56f
  loss of
    in combination syndrome, 49f

101

from hydroxyapatite in particulate solid form, 69, 69f–70f
maxillary, after implant placement, 50f
remodeling of
with Bio-Oss, 98, 98f, 99f, 100
Bio-Oss and synthetic hydroxyapatite in, 98, 99f, 99t
rabbit femur study of, 98–100
resorption lacunae in, 98, 99f
Bone formation
with Bio-Oss, 93
comparison of spongiosa and corticalis, 95, 95f, 96f
femoral, 94f, 95, 95f
lamellar, 100, 94f
rabbit study of, 96, 97f
Bone graft substitutes
characterization of, 87–88
comparison of
mercury porosimetry in, 91t
transmission electron microscopy in, 88, 89t
ideal, 87–88
material considerations in, 87
mechanical properties of, 92, 92t
Bone graft(s)
autogenous, 3–11
mechanisms of, 13–21. *See also* Conduction; Guided tissue regeneration; Induction.
sources of, 3
anterior tibia, 10
cranium, 4, 9
fibula, 9–10
ilium, 4–9. *See also* Iliac crest graft.
intraoral, 10–11
mandibular tori, 10, 10f
maxillary tuberosity, 10
mentum, 10
retromolar, 10, 11f
rib, 3–4
tibia, 3, 10
Bone interface, response around root-form implants in Bio-Oss-implanted sockets, 54, 56, 56f
Bone morphogenetic protein (BMP). *See also* Induction.
carriers for, 15f, 18
genetic engineering of, 14–15

C

Calvarial grafts, 4, 9
Cancellous bone chips, human, 89t, 91t
Canine teeth
movement of
lateral, 79, 80, 81f
medial, 79, 79f

Chrome-cobalt mesh, with PMCB and membrane barrier, in mandibular reconstruction, 19, 20f
Cleft palate. *See* Maxillary cleft(s).
Collagen sponge, as carrier for bone morphogenetic protein, 15f, 16f, 18
Combination syndrome
description of, 53
iatrogenic variation of, 50f, 53
treatment of, 53–54
bone density increase with, 54
fabrication of denture in, 50f, 53
mandible in
PMCB graft in, 53
maxilla in
PMCB graft in, 53
PMCB and Bio-Oss in titanium mesh in, 49f
prosthesis in, 54
one-stage procedure, 50f, 53
placement of abutments in, 50f, 53
Conduction
description of, 13
use of, 13–14, 14f, 15f
Connective tissue, PMCB and Bio-Oss as barrier to ingrowth of, 63f, 63–64, 64f
Cortical grafts
maxillary
dehisced, 47, 47f
nonviability of, 46f, 46–47
root-form implants in, 46f
Cortical-cancellous grafts
as strut
failure of, 75, 75f
for placement of PMCB and Bio-Oss, 58, 60f, 61f
Cranium. *See* Calvarial grafts.

E

Extraction sockets
Bio-Oss implanted
animal studies of, 51f, 53, 55f
bone density increase with, 54–55
PMCB and Bio-Oss in, 42, 44
root-form implants in, 42–45. *See also* Root-form implants, in one- and two-tooth edentulous defects.
TiMesh grid in, 44, 45f

F

Femoral cutaneous nerve paresthesia, from harvest of anterior iliac crest bone, 8
Fibula
as source of free graft, 9, 10f

Free-end saddle prosthesis, bone loss with, 53
Free-flap grafts
   in oncologic surgical defects, 67f
   in maxillary and mandibular reconstruction, 73, 73f

G

Grafts. *See* Allogeneic grafts; Alloplastic materials; Autogenous grafts; Bone grafts; Bone graft substitutes; Free-flap grafts; Particulate marrow and cancellous bone grafts; Xenogeneic grafts.
Guided tissue regeneration (osteophylic response)
   barrier membranes in
      appropriate use of, 19, 20f, 21f
   description of, 18, 18f
   exclusion of cells in, 18
Gunshot wounds
   mandibular reconstruction following
      bar prosthesis with PMCB and Bio-Oss in, 66f
      placement of PMCB and Bio-Oss in titanium mesh in, 64, 65f
      placement of root-form implants in, 65f
      prosthesis in, 65f, 66f

H

Hematoma, from harvest of iliac crest bone, 9
Hernia
   from anterior iliac crest harvest, 9
   from posterior iliac crest harvest, 8
HTR (hard-tissue replacement). See Poly(methylmethacrylate)
Hydroxyapatites, modulus of elasticity values of, 92, 92t

I

Ileus, from harvest of posterior iliac crest bone, 8
Iliac crest graft
   for cleft palate
      harvesting of, 76
      placement and closure of, 76, 77f
   as gold standard, 3
   harvesting of
      from anterior crest, 5, 6f, 7f
      complications and morbidities of, 8–9
      lateral table osteotomy in, 5, 6f, 7f, 9
      medial table approach in, 9
      from posterior crest, 5, 7f, 8f
      trephined core *versus* curettage in, 5, 6f
Induction. *See also* Bone morphogenetic protein (BMP).
   bone morphogenetic protein in, 14–17
   carriers for inductive surfaces in, 18
   demineralized freeze-dried protein in, 17
   of pluripotential cells, 4f
Infection, maxillary, titanium mesh in reconstruction following, 68f, 69
Interpore 200, 89t, 91t

M

Mandible
   atrophy of
      iliac crest cortical strut graft for
         lingual placement of, 58, 60f
         maintenance with circummandibular wires of, 58, 60f
         placement of PMCB and Bio-Oss against, 58, 60f
         treatment with PMCB and Bio-Oss of, 56, 57f
   BMP-regenerated bone in
      following hemimandibulectomy in Rhesus monkey, 15, 16f
      in Macaca fascicularis, 15, 17, 17f
   in combination syndrome
      PMCB graft in, 53
      iliac crest graft with mandibular tissue bar on IMZ implants, 58, 62f
   partially edentulous
      titanium grid mesh in, 58, 59f
   reconstruction of
      PMCB and Bio-Oss mixture in, 20, 21f
      with PMCB and membrane barrier, 19, 20f
      titanium grid mesh in, 58
      staged root-form implants in, 58, 62f
Mandibular tori, particulate cortical grafts from, 10, 109f
Maxilla
   in combination syndrome
      PMCB graft in, 53
   reconstruction of bone deficiencies in
      anterior, 32, 32f
      exposure of site in, 31
      placement of PMCB and Bio-Oss in titanium mesh for, 31f, 31–32, 32f
      preparation of cast and titanium mesh for, 29–31, 30f
      self-tapping titanium mesh screw in, 32, 32f
      titanium mesh with PMCB for, 29
Maxillary tuberosity bone graft, 10
Maxillary cleft(s)
   bilateral
      after grafting, 78, 78f
   cortical grafts in, 75
   cortical-cancellous rib graft in, 75, 75f
      history of, 75
   PMCB from iliac crest in, 76
   principles of, 75

iliac crest graft for
  harvesting of, 76
  long-term results with, 76–80
  placement of, 76, 77f
midline, 82, 84f
PMCB graft in
  alignment of teeth following, 79f, 79–80
  arch expansion following, 77–78, 78f
  follow-up of, 76
  procedures in, 76, 77f
  timing of, 80
PMCB and Bio-Oss graft in
  abutments in, 83f
  for alveolar augmentation, 80, 82, 82f
  maintenance of
    with TiMesh implant, 82, 83f
  placement of, 82, 83f
root-form implants in
  advantages of, 80
  for bilateral and unilateral clefts, 80, 81f, 82, 82f, 83f
  completed prostheses, 83f
  for midline clefts, 82, 84f, 85f
  placement of, 80–85
unilateral
  orthopedic appliance for arch expansion in, 78, 78f
Mentum bone graft, 10
Modulus of elasticity
  with Bio-Oss, 92, 92t

N

Natural bone mineral. *See* Bio-Oss.

O

Osteoblasts, induction of, 4, 4f
OsteoGen, 89t, 91t
Osteogenic precursor cells. *See* Pluripotential cells
Osteograft/N, 89t, 91t
Osteophylic response. *See* Guided tissue regeneration.

P

Particulate marrow and cancellous bone (PMCB). *See also* Autogenous grafts.
  donor sites for, 3–11,
  in maxillary clefts, 77–80. *See also* Maxillary cleft(s), PMCB graft for.
  uses of, 3, 4f
Particulate marrow and cancellous bone (PMCB) and Bio-Oss (natural bone mineral)
  as barrier to ingrowth of connective tissue, 63f, 63–64, 64f
  for conventional and implant-borne prostheses, 49, 49f, 50f
  used following bone loss from atrophy and infection, 68f, 69
  used following hemimaxillectomies and maxillary resections, 64
  used following placement of particulate solid hydroxyapatite, 69, 69f–70f
  layered placement technique for, 31, 32, 37
  in oncologic surgical defects
    mandibular, 64, 67f
    maxillary, 64
  in one- and two-tooth edentulous defects, 42, 44
  for premaxillary deficiency following comminuted fracture, 69, 71f–72f
  in reconstruction of atrophic mandible
    10-year follow-up of IMZ implants in, 58, 62f
  in reconstruction of mandible following gunshot trauma, 64, 65f, 66f, 73f
  in restoration of alveolar ridge, 56, 57f
  with TiMesh with free-flap grafts
    maxillary and mandibular, 73, 73f
Pluripotential cells, 3
  induction, 4, 4f
  location of, 3, 4f
PMCB. *See* Particulate marrow and cancellous bone.
Polyhydroxyethyl methacrylate (PHEMA) spheres (HTR)
  as carrier of bone morphogenetic protein, 15f, 18

R

Resorption, 98, 98f
Retromolar mandible, graft harvest from, 10, 11f
Root-form implants
  advantages of titanium mesh technique in, 51–52
  in cleft palate, 80, 81f, 82, 82f, 83
  in gun-shot wound defect, 65f
  integration of
    in cortical versus PMCB graft, 48, 48f
  mandibular
    staged, 58, 62f
  in one- and two-tooth edentulous defects. *See also* Extraction sockets.
    Bio-Oss only in, 43f, 44
    completed, 45f
    delayed placement of, 42, 43f
    immediate placement of, 42, 43f
    microporous filter membrane in, 44
    PMCB and Bio-Oss in, 42, 44
    screws for TiMesh grid in, 44, 45f
    special materials in, 44–45

TiMesh grid in, 44, 44f
in partially edentulous areas, 37–41
   creation of a vestibule, 39, 40f
   placement of implants, 39, 41f
   placement of titanium mesh and graft material, 37–38, 38f
   removal of titanium mesh, 38–39, 40f
PMCB *versus* solid grafts for, 46–52
   integration of root-form implants in, 48–51
   response to dehiscence and, 47, 47f
   viability of, 46–47
staged, 42, 43f, 58, 62f

S

Sartorius muscle, anterior superior iliac spine interference in, 9
Split-thickness skin graft
   for restoration of buccal vestibule, 61f
Steri-Oss implants
   in BMP-regenerated bone
      antral, 17f
      mandibular, 16f

T

Tibia
   anterior surface as PMCB donor site, 3, 5t, 10
Timing
   of bone grafting for cleft palate, 76, 80
TiMesh. *See* Titanium grid mesh; Titanium mesh.
Titanium grid mesh, 44, 44f, 45f, 46, 58, 59f. *See also* Titanium mesh.
Titanium mesh. *See also* Titanium grid mesh.
   0.015-inch thickness, 29, 44
   0.020-inch thickness, 58, 59f
   advantages of, 29, 51–52
   biocompatibility of, 25–29
   cleft palate, in treatment of, 82, 84f, 85f
   creation of vestibule with, 34–35, 38–39
   ductility and tensile strength of, 26–27
   fatigue strength of, 25
   flexible form of, 44f
   in labial plate after tooth extraction, 54
   in maxillary reconstruction, 49f, 68f, 69f, 70f, 71f, 72f
      for conventional prostheses, 29–35
      with free-flap graft, 73, 73f
      placement with graft material, 31–33, 37–38
      presurgical procedures in, 29–31
      at 10-year follow-up, 35, 35f
   in mandibular reconstruction
      with free flaps, 73
      for implant-borne prostheses, 48
      near mental foramen, 44, 45f
      following trauma, 65f, 66f, 67f
   with membrane material liner, 18f, 19
   for one- and two-tooth edentulous defects, 42, 43f
   physical properties of, 25–27, 27f
   purity of, 25–26, 27f
   removal of, 33–34, 38–39
      dissection of fibrous tissue in, 33, 33f
      incision for, 33, 33f
      suturing of palatal mucosal flap to periosteum, 33, 33f
      titanium screw removal in, 34
   rounded corners of, 25–26, 27f
      versus mesh with sharp edges, 26, 26f
   self-tapping screws with, 27f, 27-28, 32, 32f
      cross-section of, 28f
      integration with host bone, 28, 28f
      macroscopic view in place, 28f
      versus nonself-tapping, 27f, 27–28
      removal of, 34

V

Vestibular lengthening procedure
   for secondary epithelialization of maxilla
      following removal of TiMesh, 70f
      periosteum exposure, 34, 34f, 35
      ten-year postoperative view
         with dentures, 35f
         without dentures, 35f

X

Xenogeneic bone material. *See* Bio-Oss; Bone graft substitutes.
Xenogeneic grafts, 3, 87–92